Loss and Bereavement in Childbearing

Bereavement is a difficult issue for midwives to manage and families suffer when the care they receive is inadequate or inappropriate. Written by an experienced midwife and researcher, *Loss and Bereavement in Childbearing* examines ways in which midwives can assist families to embark on a healthy grieving process.

This new edition of a groundbreaking work reflects the important developments in the general understanding of and research into loss and death. Providing a wealth of information for both midwives and all concerned with childbearing, the book discusses issues such as:

- perinatal and neonatal loss
- miscarriage and termination for fetal abnormality
- maternal death
- the difficulties encountered during future childbearing
- the benefits of counselling and self-help groups
- loss in successful childbearing.

Combining an authoritative research-based orientation with a critical yet human approach to this sensitive topic, the book aids midwives in providing effective care and support to those who experience loss. This book will be of interest to both practising and student midwives as well as other health professionals, bereavement counsellors, bereavement researchers and parents.

Rosemary Mander is Professor of Midwifery at the University of Edinburgh, Scotland.

Loss and Bereavement in Childbearing

Second Edition

Rosemary Mander

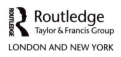

Routledge
Taylor & Francis Group

LONDON AND NEW YORK

First published 1994 by Blackwell Scientific
This edition published 2006
by Routledge
2 Park Square, Milton Park, Abingdon, Oxon, OX14 4RN

Simultaneously published in the USA and Canada
by Routledge
270 Madison Avenue, New York, NY 10016

Routledge is an imprint of the Taylor & Francis Group

© 1994, 2006 Rosemary Mander

Typeset in Goudy by RefineCatch Ltd, Bungay, Suffolk
Printed and bound in Great Britain by
TJ International Ltd, Padstow, Cornwall

British Library Cataloguing in Publication Data
A catalogue record for this book is available from the British Library

Library of Congress Cataloging in Publication Data
Mander, Rosemary
  Loss and bereavement in childbearing / Rosemary
Mander.—[New ed.]
    p. ; cm.
  Includes bibliographical references and index.
  1. Miscarriage—Psychological aspects.   2. Perinatal death—
Psychological aspects.   3. Stillbirth—Psychological aspects.   4.
Childbirth—Psychological aspects.   5. Midwifery—Psychological
aspects.   6. Bereavement—Psychological aspects.   7. Loss
(Psychology)
  1. Title.
    [DNLM: 1. Bereavement.   2. Fetal Death.   3. Abortion,
Spontaneous—psychology.   4. Attitude to Death.   5. Social
Support.   WQ 225 M272L   2005]
  RG648.M345   2005–06–01
  618.3'92—dc22
  2005014821

ISBN10: 0–415–35410–2 (hbk)
ISBN10: 0–415–35411–0 (pbk)
ISBN10: 0–203–00085–4 (eb)

ISBN13: 9–78–0–415–35410–3 (hbk)
ISBN13: 9–78–0–415–35411–0 (pbk)
ISBN13: 9–78–0–203–00085–4 (eb)

Contents

	List of figures	vii
	List of tables	viii
	Acknowledgements for the First Edition	ix
	Acknowledgements for the Second Edition	x
	Introduction	xi
1	Loss, bereavement, grief and mourning	1
2	Loss in 'successful' childbearing	13
3	Researching childbearing loss: problems, dangers and opportunities	20
4	Features of loss in childbearing	34
5	Caring for the grieving mother	58
6	Bereavement counselling	79
7	Family grief	89
8	Grief in the neonatal unit	108
9	The death of a mother	129
10	Staff reactions and support	145
11	Staff grieving and crying	165
12	Self-help support groups	179
13	Future childbearing	196
	Conclusion: benefits and meanings	207

Appendix 1 Mysterious discovery: children's cemetery has
been found in Astypalaia   210
Appendix 2 My youngest brother   211
References   213
Index   234

Figures

5.1 Photograph of a stillborn baby (1925) 68
5.2 The family of the baby in Figure 5.1 during the pregnancy 69
5.3 A contemporary photograph of a grieving mother with her stillborn baby 70
9.1 The monument to Lady Jane Crewe in Westminster Abbey, London 132

Tables

1.1   Dual process activities   8
8.1   Babies' birth weight in two studies   109
11.1   Hospital staff reports of having cried at work   168

Acknowledgements for the First Edition

I acknowledge the generous financial support provided by the Iolanthe Trust, to enable me to undertake the study mentioned in this book. I appreciate the help and support given by midwifery managers and others who helped me to gain access to suitable mothers and midwives. I am most grateful of all to the mothers and the midwives who generously gave of their experience and their expertise, their time and their tears.

I would also like to acknowledge the help of Claire Greig and of my colleagues Sarah Baggaley and Nick Watson for their comments on some of the chapters. I particularly appreciate the help of Iain Abbot, who not only read chapters, but who also helped me in other ways too numerous to recall.

Acknowledgements for the Second Edition

My gratitude to all those who contributed to the First Edition continues unabated. Additionally, I would like to thank Dr Claire Greig again, but this time for both her encouragement to produce this Second Edition and her help with Chapter 8. My thanks go to Dr Rosalind K. Marshall for all her help and support, but especially for her contribution to Chapter 9. Additionally, I would like to express my thanks to the following friends, colleagues and contacts for their input: Despoina Anagnostou; Marguerite (Peg) A. Dimarco; Dr Yvonne Freer; Leslie Ann Grout; Dr Martina Hexel; Dr Ulrich Kropiunigg; Annie Lau; Anne Robertson; Erica Stewart; Mark Squire; Professor Kristen M. Swanson; Allan Thomson; Dr Renate Wagner. Thanks also to Jenny Newland for her help in preparing the manuscript.

To Iain Abbot, I would like to add to his continuing help in ways too numerous to recall, my appreciation of his permitting me to share his personal grief.

Introduction

How do I introduce loss?

I don't think I do.

I don't need to make the introduction because you know loss already. Was it when your grandmother died? Was it when your first child was miscarried? Was it when a mother you'd been caring for had an unexpected stillbirth? Or was it when your childish idealisation of your mother was replaced by your realisation of her very real humanity? Or was it when your first 'steady' told you that they were 'chucking' you? Or was it the day you got home to find that a burglar had messed up your bedroom? Or perhaps it was when you didn't come top in the exams. Or when your partner was made redundant. Or it might have been when what your brother did to you snatched away your youthful innocence.

We all know loss. It is fundamental to life. You might say it is a fact of life. And like so many facts of life, together with the grief which follows, it allows us to grow and to develop into the people we are. Inevitably our minds home in first of all on the major losses, often of those we love. But as we have seen already there is no shortage of other examples.

It is neither easy nor necessary to separate out our personal losses from those we face in the course of our work. The painful memories which we may regard as safely out of the way have a nasty habit of reappearing at surprising and discomforting moments. In the course of my work I have certainly found that my own losses, some real and some potential, have been brought into sharper focus by my reading, writing and caring. There has been more than one occasion when I have found tears dropping on to a book or on to my computer keyboard.

Although the first edition of this book was criticised for its 'chatty' approach (Sherr, 1995b) I use the first person, because loss is so crucially personal. I make no apology for this. It serves to remind us that reading and learning are about sharing knowledge and ideas. Thus, the ideas and experience which I offer in this book interact with those of you, the reader. Although I have written this book it is not because I claim unique expertise in this area. I attempt as far as possible to avoid a prescriptive, dogmatic, 'expert' or 'cookbook' approach. Is there a recipe for effective care of a grieving mother? Like those we care for, we all have our own unique expertise. In certain situations, such as her grief, only the mother knows what it is like. Only by accepting how she sees it do we have a basis from which to begin to help her.

While recognising that our care is increasingly oriented towards the care of the family, I emphasise throughout this book our care of the mother. This is because the mother is invariably intimately involved with loss in childbearing, while others may either be less involved or else differently involved. I concentrate on her reactions and difficulties and assume that many of her feelings will be shared by those close to her. I mention other family members when they may be affected differently. It is possible that others near her, such as the father, may have similar, or perhaps even more extreme, reactions, but I address his orientation and response in Chapter 7.

My use of the word 'mother' may also be frowned on, because it may be seen as disregarding the woman's many other characteristics. I would argue, though, that, in the context of perinatal loss, the fact of her motherhood is crucially important. It is for this reason that I use 'mother' in preference to 'woman'.

I begin this book by attempting to sort out the words which are widely used in the context of loss and grief. This attempt, hopefully, lays the ground for a serious examination of the issues.

This book then continues with two chapters examining events around the time of birth when a baby is lost and when she lives. I suggest that neither is a uniformly negative or positive experience.

Because of its importance in all aspects of our work, and particularly when there is grief, the chapter on our use and misuse of research is next. In Chapter 4 we consider the ways in which loss in childbearing may manifest itself in order to set the scene for the next chapter on the principles of care. Four chapters on specific aspects of care follow: counselling, other family members, the death of a mother and the care of the family with a baby in NNU. In Chapters 10 and 11 we hold up a mirror to look at our own responses to loss. These lead us to think about another group of carers, whose input is not to be underestimated; these are the systems of lay support. Finally, we look forward to the mother's experience in any future pregnancy.

In writing this book my main aim is to help the midwife caring for a mother experiencing any form of loss in childbearing. I hope, through this book, to prevent the additional suffering which a woman may face when her carers are unable to provide appropriate care. I hope also to minimise the feelings which the midwife encounters when she knows that the care being provided is less than it should be. Although we ordinarily perceive bereavement as a totally negative event with unhealthy or unpleasant consequences, this book aims to help those involved to begin the process of grieving in the most favourable circumstances.

1 Loss, bereavement, grief and mourning

Attitudes to death have changed over the past couple of centuries. In current Western society attitudes to loss through death tend to be similar to the Victorian attitude to sex – the ultimate unmentionable. It may be that our attitudes to these two essential aspects of human life have become reversed. This is partly due to society now tending to focus more on young, healthy, sexually active people, despite our increasing population of elderly people. Because of this altered focus and the changing pattern of health and illness, the spectre of death is no longer our constant companion. It may be as a result that these two taboos have become transposed (Gorer, 1965).

Despite these changing attitudes, the fact remains that death is still a fundamental part of life. Our grief over the loss of a loved one is the price that we must pay for the pleasure which that love brought; 'we cannot fully know the rich textured experience of being alive until we learn to look calmly into the face of death' (Campbell, 1979).

The reality and proximity of loss are demonstrated by the need, in order to grow and develop into mature human beings, to progress through certain phases involving the loss of aspects of our earlier selves. These aspects include the loss of our childhood selves, our fantasy parents, our youthful expectations and the world as we have known it. Each loss requires to be mourned, at least momentarily, in order to recognise its passage and prepare to move on to the next phase in our lives.

The inevitability of death still tends to be avoided, if not ignored, although the topic is now being opened up, especially by researchers and other writers. It may be that, as the population becomes older, death in old age is becoming a more widely recognised and more easily accepted event. Whether this acceptance applies to loss and death at the opposite end of the age range is less certain.

Words and meanings

Our understanding of the experience of the person who has been bereaved has grown vastly over the past half-century. This growth has been due largely to the interest of researchers and other workers from a wide range of disciplines, including psychology, physiology, psychiatry and sociology, as well as nursing and midwifery. Such a heterogeneous input into our knowledge-base provides, not only a more comprehensive picture of this experience, but also a greater diversity in the meanings linked to the fundamental terms. Because of this diversity and for the sake of clarity, I begin by exploring the meanings of these terms as I use them.

Grief

Although it may have many social, financial and practical as well as other implications, the essence of the experience of loss lies in the person's psychological, affective or emotional response (Weston *et al.*, 1998: 259). This is grief. It is quite specific, as well as being intensely personal and individual. These aspects, though, must not be allowed to distract our attention from both the complexity of this emotion and the depth of the person's feelings. The scope of grief may be broadened marginally by including in it those behaviours which are directly associated. Thus, weeping and appetite loss may be regarded as crucial parts of grief.

Grieving

As I show later in this chapter, the way in which a person's grief develops has come to underpin our knowledge of this area. The changes or developments in the person's emotional state are known, with our increasing understanding, as grieving or the grieving process.

Mourning

Grief and grieving focus solely and narrowly on the person's emotional state, albeit with a few closely associated behaviours. Mourning, however, includes the wide-ranging, more socially oriented manifestations of loss. It is through mourning that we are able to begin unravelling the psychological bonds that have cemented our relationships with those who have died. Many of the rituals or rites of passage associated with loss are culturally determined, varying according to the ethnic origin, socio-economic class, prevailing social attitudes and religious persuasion of the bereaved. The extent to which mourning reflects different grieving patterns among various cultures was researched by Cowles (1996). This study comprised several focus groups involving people from specific cultural backgrounds. Cowles showed that, unsurprisingly, mourning behaviour does vary between groups. She went on to demonstrate, however, that the personal experience of grief does not differ in any way that may be attributed to cultural heritage or ethnicity alone.

Mourning provides an opportunity for the expression of respect for the one who is lost. It also shows the sorrow of the community and support for those most intimately affected by the loss. Thus, as Clark (1991) states, mourning serves to confirm the relationships between those who remain. In this way it strengthens the continuing bonds of affection. Clark goes on to suggest that mourning rituals assist each of us to anticipate our own death, more confident in the knowledge that our dying will be recognised in a similar way.

The rituals of mourning feature changes in the appearance of mourners. In terms of clothing, this means wearing appropriate colours or items not usually worn, such as hats, armbands or black ties. There may be conventions concerning behaviour, such as standing still as the cortege passes or driving slowly behind it. The funeral and, possibly, the wake provide an opportunity for a more social form of support. The duration and expression of mourning may be rigidly culturally determined.

The implications of culture in the context of perinatal loss are becoming apparent in a finding on the small Greek island of Astypalaia. A cemetery for newborn babies, possibly dating from 750 BC (Hillson, 2002), has been found to contain the remains of about 500 babies. Archaeologists are investigating this graveyard in an effort to identify the reason for this sad assembly (Anagnostou, 2004, Appendix 1).

Bereavement

For all of us the term 'bereavement' carries a powerful connotation of the fact of loss through death. Although we accept this definition, we should bear in mind the other meanings which do not necessarily involve death. It may be that the emphasis should be on 'the fact', rather than 'death'. The other meanings of 'bereavement' become apparent through the etymological evidence. The active verb 'to bereave' means 'to steal anything of value'. From this is derived the widely used adjective 'bereft', which is the passive form of the verb; it clearly indicates the feelings of the bereaved person following various forms of loss which may be more or less tangible. Both forms are related to the verb 'to reave' (as in the 'border rievers'), meaning 'to plunder or rob'. Again, these are words which may be very appropriate to describe the feelings of a person who has been bereaved.

Loss

This term is widely used for a number of reasons. The first reason is that it indicates the 'innocence' or non-contributory involvement of the bereaved person. She has been passive in the event and is suffering through no fault of her own and is, thus, deserving of others' care and support. The word 'loss' may become particularly helpful in the later stages of grieving when the bereaved person is feeling guilty about any action or inaction on her part which she feels may have contributed to this event. 'Loss' is also a useful word because it is non-specific and may be used in a wide range of situations when grieving is the appropriate response. This word does not necessarily indicate that a death has occurred, but may suggest that the relationship with a person or an object has been altered in some other way or it may even be appropriate when some part of the body has been removed. I consider some of these other forms of loss later (please see Chapter 3).

On the other hand, it has been suggested that the term 'loss' may be less than helpful because of the other connotations which it conveys. These may be carried over from its use in other situations when it implies carelessness, verging on irresponsibility, in not taking care of one's property and allowing it to 'go missing'. Thus, this term may be seen to imply that the person who is bereaved is really at fault or is to be blamed in some other way.

Understanding meanings

The possibility of this adverse interpretation of 'loss' is one example which shows the importance of the words which we may use unthinkingly; they may give rise to unnecessary and unintended hurt in sensitive situations. 'Loss' is an example which clearly demonstrates the need to be particularly thoughtful in our communicating, particularly with those who are bereaved.

There are other, perhaps more hurtful, words which those who are bereaved may encounter in their contacts with midwives and others. As with so many occupational groups, those who work in maternity care have developed their own jargon language which serves, among other purposes, to facilitate quick, effective communication among people working under pressure. Unfortunately this jargon may be unthinkingly used in other, non-interprofessional, situations. In these circumstances the words' jargon meanings may be less than clear to the lay person, the patient or the parents. Even more seriously, the jargon may carry completely different and possibly negative meanings to the non-professional. A very apposite example in this context is the word 'abortion', which carries to a lay person the implication of deliberate interference to end a pregnancy. To health professionals, though, this term is value-free in that it means simply that the pregnancy is ending, for an unspecified reason, before the baby is viable. While a recent audit found that women now rarely encounter terms such as 'abortion' and 'blighted ovum', the words 'products of conception' continue to feature (SPCERH, 2003). It is encouraging to note that more sensitive words, such as 'miscarriage', are now used more frequently in this context, although even this term may not be devoid of negative connotations.

Although not necessarily hurtful, I avoid using the word 'fetus' in this book. It has long been known that by eight to twelve weeks the mother perceives her developing baby to have become a real person (Lumley, 1979). The use of words such as 'fetus' is not helpful to communication and may even be counterproductive in caring situations.

I have used the word 'understanding' in the sense of being aware of the issues relating to the experience of bereavement. Thus, it is being used in general terms to reflect our knowledge of this area. Although it may be well meant, it may not be helpful to say to a person who has been bereaved 'I understand how you're feeling'. This statement, while intended to reassure and comfort, serves to diminish the essentially personal nature of grief. My own experience of a well-intentioned colleague saying this to me when my father died is still disquieting. My recollection of her assumption of similarity between her father's death and that of my own father always brings back my difficulty in communicating with my father and my inability to help him to cope with the last of a long series of difficult experiences.

Meaning and caring

While considering the most appropriate words to describe the feelings and experience of the mother whose baby has died or has been lost in some other way, we should contemplate the words which we use to describe this mother. Long gone are the days when we described a mother in terms of 'the SVD in bed 4' or 'the caesarean in room 12'. These terms reduced the mother to little more than her bed or room number and carried no recognition of the person occupying that space.

One issue that arises when we contemplate what to call her is whether she should be 'a woman' or 'a mother'. For most childbearing women the term 'mother' serves to reduce them to only one of a multiplicity of characteristics. In the present context, though, there are good reasons for addressing and referring to this woman as a 'mother'. That she is a mother is not in doubt and much of our care revolves around helping her, despite having no baby with her, to realise this. Is it appropriate to refer to this woman as 'a grieving mother'? This term is widely and sympathetically used, but we need to question the effect it has on our perception of her. It, perhaps correctly, focuses our attention on what we consider to be the feature of her care which is most deserving of our attention. Unfortunately, though, it ignores the fact that she is a complete person with, simultaneously, a wide range of other feelings and needs. As long ago as 1985, Gohlish showed that the mother without a baby has the difficulties and discomforts which many new mothers encounter, such as relationship adjustments, a sore perineum, afterpains or painful breasts, as well as the infinitely more difficult task of coping with the loss of her baby. It is essential for us to regard this mother as a complete person who has been bereaved and who needs care which takes many forms, and not only help her with her grieving, crucial though that help may be. In making this plea for the holistic care of this mother, I accept that we are all too often accused of ignoring the emotional and spiritual aspects of care. On this occasion, however, I find myself reversing the usual plea to recommend that the physical and practical aspects of this mother's care should be given the attention they deserve.

Healthy grieving

In the context of dying and death the concept of a 'good death' is becoming recognised (Thoresen, 2003; Fisher, 2001; Smith, 2003), although its precise nature may be determined by a range of cultural and other factors (Walter, 2003). The value of this concept is not easy to assess because it may be criticised for providing little more than an intellectualisation of an essentially emotional experience. Despite this criticism, I suggest that the early stages of healthy grieving may be facilitated by appropriate care. Grieving has been shown by research (see page 7) to involve the development of the person's emotional state, from the initial numbing impact of learning of the loss, through to the point where memories may be recalled with equanimity. The role of the midwife is to help the mother to begin this process of adjusting to the situation in which she finds herself. While accepting that bereavement cannot be regarded as anything other than painful, the midwife is in a position to enable the mother to create memories which she will eventually be able to recall with some degree of satisfaction. This means that she will be able to bring to mind events around the birth and conclude 'Yes, we did that right' or 'I'm glad we were able to do that for my baby' or 'I can look back now and know I was happy with most of the care I received'.

In her care the midwife is able to establish the foundations of healthy grieving. These will end, in due course, with the resolution of the mother's grief and the associated personal growth. The mother will eventually come to realise that her loss has a less negative side and that, as Parkes (1996) observed, 'The experience of grieving can strengthen and bring maturity to those who have been protected from misfortune.'

Grief and grieving theory

The conceptualisation of grief has evolved alongside other psychosociobiological ideas over the past century. These ideas may be classified according to their origins.

Psychoanalytic theory, derived from the Freudian views of mourning, was a crucial influence on later developments (Freud 1955 [1893–95]). The understanding of grief in this context, though, has been limited by the poor differentiation between case studies and therapeutic interventions.

'**Grief work**' is an enduring concept which emerged out of the groundbreaking research by Lindemann (1944). This unprecedented study followed a tragic fire in the Cocoanut Grove night club in Boston, Massachusetts in 1942. Lindemann is credited with having been the first to introduce this concept. Through it he indicated that grieving is not static, but an active process in which the ability of the person to complete their task is a major factor affecting the duration and nature of their grief.

The **stages of grieving,** described by Kübler-Ross (1970), built on Lindemann's view of active grief. Kübler-Ross's work was based on her study of people facing death. These well-known and generally accepted stages feature (1) denial or isolation, (2) confusion or anger, (3) bargaining, (4) depression, and (5) acceptance. The concept of stages is valuable in that it emphasises the dynamic nature of grieving as well as the crucially active role of the bereaved person. A serious disadvantage of Kübler-Ross's work, though, is that this descriptive concept may become prescriptive if a 'professional' considers that grieving 'ought' to progress in a certain pre-ordained sequence. This prescriptiveness may arouse unnecessary and counterproductive anxiety. Such an approach also has the potential for limiting individual variability.

Attachment theory combines the work of a number of late-twentieth-century psychologists whose work is loosely related to the developmental theories of Piaget (Wood, 1998). The pioneering work of John Bowlby (1961) indicated that attachment serves as a biological mechanism which protects the individual, in order to ensure the survival of both the individual and the species. Bowlby's observations of children separated from and reunited with their mothers (see Chapter 2) established a typical response in the child to the threat and insecurity which such a loss carried. Bowlby's work may be criticised on a number of grounds, including the tenuous link between childhood separation and bereaved people. Thus, his fundamental tenet, that the reason for grief is to cut the bond with the dead person, is open to question (see 'Biography' p. 8).

Colin Murray Parkes (1987) applied Bowlby's ideas on attachment in his work with women who had been widowed. This work resulted in astute descriptions of the emotional, behavioural and physical manifestations of the women's grief.

Dual process theory arose out of observation of the variation between individuals in the duration and progress of grieving, as well as people's tendency to oscillate and hesitate between stages (Parkes, 1996; Stroebe and Schut, 1995). These variations have been related to gender differences (see Chapter 7). This oscillation may be seen as exemplifying the movement between the more 'feminine' or passive style of grieving, which is combined sequentially with the more active or 'masculine' style. These researchers argue that, rather than being purely gender-linked and clearly differentiated, these styles or processes combine in any one individual, irrespective of their gender. This interpretation of coping with grief features a range of both 'female' loss-oriented activities and a range of 'male' restoration-oriented activities. A combination of these strategies may be employed by the grieving person in their attempts to resolve the pain of loss. Examples of the two types of activities are shown in Table 1.1.

In this way the nature of grief, which has traditionally been regarded as a dichotomy between the passive feminine and the active masculine, is being reinterpreted more as a dialectic between two distinct coping styles. In order to understand a person's grieving, the dual process theory relates their grief to the position on the trajectory of grief rather than to their gender. In the context of this theoretical background Thompson (1997) argues that

Table 1.1. Dual process activities

Loss oriented activities	Restoration oriented activities
(stereotypically female)	(stereotypically male)
grief work	denial/avoidance
facing grief	broken ties/bonds
breaking bonds/ties	controlled distraction
approach	doing other things
intrusion	suppression

oscillation is not only healthy in grieving, but that it is also crucial. He maintains that neither the loss-oriented activities nor the restoration-oriented activities *alone* facilitate healthy grief.

Biography has been advanced by Walter (1999) to contradict the prevailing view that the bereaved must completely detach themselves from their memories of the dead in order to 'let go' and move on in life. This reaction to Bowlby's orthodoxy (see page 21) resonates with a similar North American process (Silverman and Klass, 1996). The purpose of 'biography' is to integrate the dead person, by finding a psychological place for the memories of them in the continuing life. The biography is achieved by conversation about the dead person by those acquainted with her. The acceptance of biography has been facilitated by consumerism, questioning of so-called 'experts', postmodern diversity and increasing acceptance of spiritual phenomena.

A general pattern of grief

What may be called a 'general pattern' of grieving is common to the various models described in the literature. Each researcher/author, though, emphasises different aspects, depending on the sample on whom they focused (the bereaved or the dying) and the intended audience (producing a more or less complex model). We need to approach the concept of a 'general pattern' with caution. It is not possible to assume that those involved in the research studies from which this pattern is drawn were representative of all grieving people or that the findings are generally applicable.

The immediate reaction comprises a temporary defence mechanism consisting essentially of delaying tactics which serve to insulate the bereaved person from the unacceptable reality of death (Engel, 1961). This allows time for rallying her emotional resources in preparation for the eventual realisation. When the delaying tactics end, the bereaved person begins to accept the reality of the loss. Somatic symptoms such as sighing respirations may be evident. This first stage has been described in various ways. Jones explains it in terms of shock (1989), suggesting a physiological response with or without psychological connotations and the possibility of pathological developments. Kübler-Ross assumed a more purely psychological approach when she described this first stage as denial. In his account of defence and searching, Parkes emphasises the need of the bereaved person to protect herself from the awful reality and implies a tentative movement towards the acceptance of that reality.

Developing awareness gradually manifests itself. With the dawning realisation of the loss come the initial, powerful emotional responses (Engel, 1961). Guilt, associated with concern about unfinished business, may be a major feature. Anger directed at a wide range of probably innocent people demonstrates a partial awareness of the reality of the loss. The need to search for the one who is lost reflects the preoccupation with the physical absence of the dead person. This search may be aggravated by perceptions involving various senses, sometimes known as hallucinations, indicating the presence of the person who is lost. Examples would include the mother feeling her baby moving within her or hearing her baby crying. Bargaining permits a gradual, controlled realisation combined with excuse-making in an attempt to rationalise the loss. As each of these emotional responses is found to be a less than adequate solution it gives way to aimlessness, despondency and apathy which has been termed 'disorganisation' (Bowlby, 1961) and which heralds the onset of the ultimate despair associated with complete recognition of the loss.

Full realisation is demonstrated by the profound depression mentioned by Jones, Kübler-Ross and Parkes. The recognition of the loss may be transferred onto the body of the bereaved person as feelings of bodily mutilation, such as the 'great emptiness' mentioned by a widow (Parkes, 1976). This depression brings with it psychological changes, such as poor concentration and difficulty in sleeping, as well as bodily problems such as those affecting the gastro-intestinal tract.

Resolution is the final stage of grieving, which is said to have been achieved when the bereaved person is able to remember comfortably, realistically and with equanimity the pleasures and disappointments of their lost relationship. Kübler-Ross describes this stage in relatively passive terms as 'acceptance', whereas Parkes describes the more active processes of recovery, reorganisation and reintegration. The extent to which this resolution depends on a severance of the emotional bonds with the dead person is still a matter of debate (Walter, 1999).

The potential for long-term personal benefit associated with bereavement is suggested in the account of the resolution stage given by Jones. He looks forward to the new identity assumed by the bereaved person. This incorporates all that has been learned from being bereaved, including the inevitable personal growth and development as well as the valuing of others' support. Both of these facilitate an increased ability to cope with other, unknown crises yet to be faced.

Variations in the usual pattern

It is crucial to recognise the variation between individuals in the duration and progress of grieving, as people oscillate and hesitate between stages. Parkes summarises the tendency towards a sequential recovery through the emergence of succeeding stages: 'Grief is not a set of symptoms which start after a loss and then gradually fade away. It involves a succession of clinical pictures which blend into and replace one another.'

Pathological forms of grief

In the same way as accounts of the stages of grieving vary, descriptions of the complicated or otherwise pathological forms of grief vary similarly. The pathological forms of grief are usually described as involving deviations in the severity of grieving and/or its duration. This observation applies to the account by Parkes which focused on the temporal aspects. On this occasion he described prolonged grieving which may occur either with or without delayed grieving.

Lindemann provided a valuable account of what he identified as 'morbid grief reactions'. He first described temporal deviations in terms of delay in beginning grieving. He then went on to detail the 'distorted' reactions including:

- overactivity without sense of loss
- hypochondriasis, involving developing the symptoms of the person who is lost
- genuine psychosomatic disorders
- changed relationships
- furious hostility
- schizophrenic picture
- withdrawal from the community and loss of social interaction
- behaviour detrimental to the person's own social and economic existence
- agitated depression.

Parkes mentions what appears to be a voluntary or deliberate deviation from the usual pattern, when he details 'excessive avoidance of grieving'. This is clearly delayed grieving, but it is a form in which the bereaved person assumes control over the timing of their grief. Parkes goes on to describe chronic grieving and also the condition termed 'hypochondriasis' by Lindemann.

Criticism of presenting an oversimplistic view of complicated grief has been levelled at Lindemann and others who followed in his footsteps. This may be ameliorated by carers focusing on, not just the person's current grieving, but also the events which preceded the grief and even the loss. That is, it may be necessary to take account of the relationship between the bereaved person and the one for whom they are grieving. Knowledge of the relationship permits, according to Rynearson (1982), categorisation of a dysfunctional grief response:

- **Dependent grief syndrome** involves an imbalanced relationship in which the bereaved person has been and continues to be clinging and over-reliant on the person who is lost.
- **Unexpected loss syndrome** perpetuates the initial shock and denial response in a long-term withdrawn anxiety state.
- **Conflicted grief syndrome** is associated with an ambivalent relationship, whose uncertain nature may delay the onset of grieving.

Rynearson explains how this approach to pathologic forms of grief may be utilised in the care of people whose grieving is dysfunctional. This approach emphasises, in perinatal loss, that the midwife and other carers should avoid making assumptions about the feelings of the mother for the baby and that grieving will follow a prescribed pattern. Such assumptions may not, according to Rynearson, facilitate grieving.

Unique features of perinatal loss

In order to refute her argument, Rosanne Cecil (1996) suggests that perinatal loss has limited impact because there is no birth of a new or death of an old person. The impact on those involved is that, like any form of loss, it presents difficulties in adjustment. Loss around the time of birth, however, carries with it certain problems which may serve to confound the progress of healthy grieving. As midwives we must be especially aware of the possibility of these problems and intervene appropriately to prevent their occurrence and facilitate grieving.

The horror, which death and loss inevitably carry with them, is particularly acute for the new mother. Being young, her experience of previous loss, if any, is limited. For some mothers, their adolescent adjustments are barely completed; even less have they acquired the maturity needed to come to terms with loss and death (Bourne, 1979). This sense of horror is aggravated by the not entirely inappropriate emphasis our society places on the healthiness or normality of childbearing. While the general media emphasise the physiological nature of childbearing, little attention is given to the possibility of what may be known as 'reproductive failure'. This serves to increase the mother's difficulty in accepting the situation when it arises.

In spite of the prevalent perception of the normality of childbearing, it remains imbued with some magical, almost mystical, qualities. This awe is often impressed on me by mothers admiring their newborn babies who ask 'Did she really come out of me?' It may be that the removal of childbirth from the domestic setting to the hospital has served to increase this sense of wonder and to hinder the acceptance of any deviation in this process.

The bewilderment which follows the simultaneous occurrence of new life and death relates to the general assumption that there will be a life-span, supposedly three score years and ten, separating the two events. When new life and death appear to become fused together, our entire perception of the world may be called into question. As Bourne states, 'the experience becomes one that stands reality on its head' (1979). This point is raised in McHaffie's useful summary of the features of parental loss, along with 'loss of future', 'failure to protect', 'loss of role' and 'unseen loss' (2001: 6).

If the baby has some unexpected kind of malformation, the mother may encounter even greater challenges in recognising the baby to whom she has given birth as the one she had been expecting. This may be especially hard for the mother who assumes that the battery of prenatal tests had given her baby a 'clean bill of health'.

The difficulties experienced by those caring for the mother may aggravate her difficulty in coming to terms with her loss. Nurses and others who come into maternity care assuming it to be a happy area of care become profoundly shocked when they realise that this is not invariably so. Their sense of having failed the mother may impede their ability to share or at least listen to her expression of her feelings of loss. The response of the staff to perinatal loss is implicit in the care of this mother and may be manifested in apparently well-meaning help, such as lone accommodation in the maternity unit and early transfer home (Hughes, 1987). The extent to which the emotional responses of staff affect their ability to provide appropriate care is discussed in Chapter 10.

The social support, essential to healthy grieving, may be less easily available to the mother who miscarries or gives birth to a stillborn baby, because her baby was not known to others near her (Lovell, 1997). Their expectations of their grandchild, for example, may help them to offer some sympathy, but not the depth of feeling shared over the loss of a known and beloved person. This problem applies to a lesser extent to the partner of the mother who is bereaved and to a greater extent if the loss occurs earlier in pregnancy.

Summary

The need of the mother for expert help and support in emotional, psychological and physical terms may be illustrated by an analogy first used by Engel. He compared the psychological trauma involved in grief with the physical trauma of a cut to the skin. He explained how healing is necessary for both forms of trauma to enable the body and mind to regain their usual balance. This process may be known as homeostasis. The degree of help needed for healing varies, depending on a number of factors. Minor abrasions normally heal spontaneously, without outside intervention, but major wounds require additional assistance. The major psychological trauma of grief following perinatal loss may also require assistance. The midwife has the earliest opportunity to provide that assistance; hopefully she also has the skill.

2 Loss in 'successful' childbearing

Even in the experiences of childbearing which we regard as ideal, when a satisfied mother produces a healthy baby, there may be an element of regret giving rise to the need to grieve. In this chapter, before moving on to focus on perinatal loss, we are thinking about the processes which ordinarily happen around the time of the birth and which may influence the mother's relationship with her baby. These processes and the loving relationship which they engender are fundamental to our understanding of loss, and the grief which is the price which we have to pay for the experience of loving (see Chapter 1). After considering the ideal childbearing situations, it is necessary to move on to those experiences which, although healthy in physical terms, leave the woman feeling traumatised. This is the woman who may find herself grieving the birth experience which she was prevented from achieving.

Attachment

Because, in developmental terms, the human baby is born at a relatively immature stage, she depends on care by others for her survival. How her care and, hence, the survival of the human species is ensured has long been a topic for speculation. Our current thinking has developed markedly since, but probably originated with, the psychoanalytic ideas of Freud. He proposed that human babies are born with innate biological drives which demand gratification; feeding is a significant example. The behaviourists' ideas followed and are closely related to Freud's, but they focused on attachment developing through reinforcement of learning. Their biological explanations were modified when in the 1960s other external factors were found to affect the mother–child relationship. A classical experiment showed that laboratory monkeys preferred the comfort of a 'cloth mother' to a 'wire mother' in a stressful situation, even though the 'wire mother' incorporated a feeding device (Harlow and Harlow, 1966).

Simultaneously in Europe, ethology (the study of animals in their natural environment) was developing. 'Imprinting' was added to our understanding of the mother–child relationship. This is the process by which, typically, a newly hatched duck assumes that the first moving object it sees is its source of comfort and security; this object would ordinarily be its mother or 'primary caregiver'. Imprinting operates only within a limited time-span, known as the critical or sensitive period (Mussen *et al.*, 1990: 157).

Ethology was integrated with psychoanalytic principles by John Bowlby (1958) to support his thesis that attachment derives from neither drive-reduction nor prior learning. He argued that a human newborn is programmed to emit signals or behaviours which will keep her caregivers sufficiently near to meet her needs and ensure her survival.

He has defined attachment as:

> any form of behaviour that results in a person attaining or retaining proximity to some other differentiated and preferred individual, who is usually conceived as stronger and/or wiser. While especially evident during early childhood, attachment behaviour is held to characterise human beings from the cradle to the grave.
>
> (Bowlby, 1984: 27–8)

Three types of newborn behaviour which initiate and maintain attachment to the caregiver have been identified (Brazelton, 1973). First, 'mutuality' indicates the reciprocity crucial to attachment. Second, 'signalling behaviours' elicit reciprocal interest through crying, vocalising and facial expressions. Third, 'executive behaviours' maintain reciprocal interaction, through activities such as rooting, sucking or grasping.

Bowlby's thesis is that attachment derives from the need for security and safety and that the young form enduring attachments with a limited number of individuals (1977). The role of attachment in healthy development lies in its provision of a secure base from which a young child is able to explore her surroundings, physically, psychologically and emotionally, and to which she may retreat if any threat becomes overwhelming (Bowlby, 1990).

Attachment and loss

Attachment is significant in the context of perinatal loss because grieving is the inevitable eventual corollary of any warm loving relationship. These two contrasting aspects of attachment became apparent in Bowlby's research with toddlers separated from their mothers. This research has been appropriately criticised because the separation was by the rather unusual process of admission to residential care. Bowlby identified a characteristic biphasic response involving protest and despair following separation, which could continue alternating for days. Eventually memory of the mother appeared to fade so that, when reunited, the child was unresponsive. As the unresponsiveness diminished it was replaced by intense emotional displays and tantrums at any temporary separation. It became apparent that the absence of the known attachment object meant that the secure base no longer existed, giving rise to terror of the unknown. Bowlby (1990) regards grief as an adult form of separation anxiety, in which the security of a known and loved person/ relationship is lost, leaving a frighteningly incomprehensible void.

Bonding

'Bonding' as a topic tends to generate more heat than light. It is the preliminary stage in the events which lead to attachment (Mussen *et al.*, 1990). The plethora of research in this area has been associated with many changes in our care of the new mother and baby. Whether these changes are necessarily for the benefit of the mother–infant dyad is questioned (Herbert and Sluckin, 1985: 123). Considerable attention has been given to early postnatal bonding because it equates with the 'love at first sight' which has commonly been assumed to be fundamental to mother-love, but events during pregnancy may be more significant in the context of perinatal loss.

Changes in pregnancy

Traditionally, we have assumed that the mother did not begin to love her baby until she laid eyes on her (Morrin, 1983). Hence, only recently has research attention been given to the process by which the mother comes to know and love her baby prenatally.

On the basis of interviews with twenty mothers whose newborn babies had died, Kennell and colleagues (1970) were able to conclude that an affectionate mother–child relationship was present by the time the baby was due to be born. As many of the mothers had had no visual or tactile contact with their babies, any postnatal stimuli to affection were excluded.

The way in which the mother's affection for her child develops has been measured using Cranley's maternal–fetal adaptation scale (MFAS) by Grace (1989). This study clearly showed the mother's increasingly positive feelings as her pregnancy progresses. The MFAS was also used to study the effects of maternal age, the experience of quickening and the physical symptoms of pregnancy on the developing relationship in eighty pregnant women (Lerum and Lobiondo-Wood, 1989). These researchers found that, while the other two factors had no impact, quickening has a positive effect on the relationship. The effects of ultrasound scans (USS), which have been said to enhance the relationship, were unclear but those mothers who were well supported showed a high level of attachment.

Whereas the two previous studies utilised a Likert-type scale, Boris *et al.* (1999) based their study of the prenatal mother–baby relationship on the mother's interpretation of fetal movements. This work showed that mothers have sufficiently clear ideas about their baby's temperament during pregnancy to complete a questionnaire anticipating how she would react in given circumstances. It is impossible to judge whether the mother's interpretations of fetal behaviour relate to her own fantasies or to the actual movements, but the researchers correctly link her interpretation to the developing relationship.

In her qualitative study, Stainton (1990) sought twenty-six couples' impressions of their unborn babies in the third trimester. She identified four different levels of awareness of the fetus, coexisting simultaneously. In ascending order of perception, Stainton described the idea of the fetus, awareness of her presence, awareness of her specific behaviours and awareness of her interactive ability. These interpretations of fetal behaviour suggest that knowledge of the psychosocial interaction with the fetus may have implications for our care in the same way as the more widely used objective assessments. This is because, as Stainton states, a stronger mother–baby relationship during pregnancy facilitates postnatal mothering.

Also tending to question the benefits of USS in enhancing the relationship, Reading (1989) reverts to attributing greater importance to quickening and recognising the autonomous nature of the fetus. Similarly, the place of USS in the developing relationship is questioned in the work of Lumley (Ewigman *et al.*, 1993). She maintains that USS have no effect after quickening and that any beneficial effects on maternal health behaviour are short-lived. Scans are associated with a number of problems, such as the lack of feedback about results which allows any anxiety engendered to persist; other problems include misdiagnosis and the indecipherability of structures seen. Lumley suggests that this 'diagnostic toxicity' (1990) deserves closer study before these investigations become yet more widely used. She questions our assumption that scans really do enhance the relationship, or whether they, like other forms of prenatal diagnosis, just 'alter the mother's clock'.

As our knowledge of the mother–baby relationship during pregnancy is still so limited, we should be wary of attempting to intervene to influence its development, as may happen postnatally. What is in little doubt, though, is the strength of the mother's relationship with her unborn baby, resulting in the need to grieve if the baby is lost.

Postnatal bonding

The research project which is best known and has probably had the greatest influence on our care of the newborn and her mother is the work by Klaus and Kennell (1976). Their experimental study was undertaken against a background of restricted mother–baby contact in USA maternity units. The control group of fourteen mothers was permitted the usual contact with their babies, that is, thirty minutes at feeding times five times per day. The experiment or extended contact (EC) group of fourteen mothers cuddled their naked babies in bed with them for an extra five hours on each of their three days in hospital. Observations and interviews were made at one month and one year.

Findings of differences between the two groups were emphasised, although there were also many similarities. During a paediatric examination, the EC women showed greater reluctance to leave their babies. The EC mothers responded more to their babies' crying and maintained greater eye contact during feeds. These researchers concluded that extended contact was necessary for bonding. Others built on this rather flimsy foundation and went as far as to suggest that, without this contact, adverse outcomes such as child abuse were more likely. In this way bonding theory evolved into dogma or bonding doctrine (Herbert and Sluckin, 1985).

This, albeit rather questionable, study has influenced our care for the better. In my experience, the requirement for the baby to be transferred to the postnatal ward within ten minutes of birth was soon abandoned. It has also influenced our care in other ways. In another unit I, as a midwife, was required to record whether a mother and baby had 'bonded' in the birthing room. A negative observation triggered social work intervention.

Whether the changes in our practice are justified by the results of this study continues to be questioned on methodological grounds. Observer bias was a problem. But it is hard to envisage how a 'blind' study of attachment could be designed, as mothers and carers must know the woman's allocation and be influenced in their behaviour and observations respectively. The sample comprised disadvantaged mothers in whom, Hawthorne-like, any intervention might have improved the outcomes.

These researchers' use of biological terms to explain their conclusions, such as 'sensitive period', ignored current knowledge of the complexity of mother–child interactions and the uniquely human social organisation. The sensitive period is implausible in humans, due to maternal mortality and morbidity requiring 'adoption' by other carers in the former and a longer and more variable attachment period in the latter.

The bonding doctrine may be further criticised for the risk of bonding publicity causing the mother to develop excessively high expectations. Failure to achieve any part of the doctrine leaves her disappointed in her experience and, more importantly, anxious about her ability to relate to her new baby. Such unrealistic expectations may be prevented by informing mothers of research evidence which indicates that attachment is a gradual process developing through knowledge of another person rather than an instantaneous all-or-nothing phenomenon.

The perfect baby

The baby on whom the mother focuses her fantasies during pregnancy is the baby she comes to love at that time. This baby's image is a composite of those she loves and admires, including herself, partner, parents and other children. If she has no children already, she will base her fantasies on what she learns from others who have children and from the media. As well as helping her to form a relationship with her baby, these fantasies enable her to work through old conflicts, especially any concerning her relationship with her own mother. Inevitably the mother's fantasies involve wishing for and dreaming of a perfect baby, but lurking in the background is the fear of a baby being born with a disability.

There is always some discrepancy between the mother's fantasies and her actual baby; she may have expected her baby to have more hair, or be surprised at how long her baby spends awake, or perhaps she had expected her baby to be a different sex. The mother's narcissistic investment in her fantasy baby (see Chapter 4) may aggravate the discrepancy between the two babies. Disentangling this discrepancy and accepting the real baby is one of the developmental tasks involved in becoming a mother.

The fantasy baby is explained by Lewis (1976, 1979a) as her 'inside baby' in contrast to her 'outside baby' for whom she must eventually care. Lewis describes the perplexing sense of loss which a mother ordinarily experiences at losing her 'inside baby', but she is consoled by the presence of her 'outside baby'. The effort which the mother needs to make to match up her fantasy baby to her real baby is neither easy nor spontaneous (Raphael-Leff, 1993) and may account for some mothers' overwhelming indifference on first seeing their baby.

The woman's experience

As well as the mother's expectations of her baby giving her at least momentary cause for regret, it is necessary to contemplate the woman's reaction to her experience of giving birth. In their research on the woman's feeling of being in control of her birth experience, Green and Baston (2003) identified the difficulty which women encounter when they feel unable to influence what staff do *to* them. This disappointment is particularly acute in first-time mothers. These findings resonate powerfully with those of McCourt and Pearce, whose study focused on ethnic minority women and who reported the experience of being 'talked *at* rather than *with*' (2000: 151). These researchers have addressed the disappointed expectations of women with uncomplicated childbearing experiences.

The problems of women whose expectations of healthy, satisfying childbearing deteriorate into a complicated or traumatic experience are different. While the need for the woman to grieve for her unfulfilled expectations would be understandable, her reaction has been addressed more in terms of the possibility or likelihood of post traumatic stress disorder (PTSD). Previous work in this area was brought together by the groundbreaking research project by Menage (1993). Although this research involved the use of a volunteer sample, Menage was able to identify the obstetric and gynaecological procedures which are likely to be followed by PTSD. These procedures may seem relatively trivial to a professional health care provider, including cervical smear, induction of labour and IUCD removal. Probably equally importantly, Menage identified the factors which aggravated the perception of trauma, such as the attendant being male and the existence of a sexual component. This research found that, as mentioned above, the woman's perception of control is fundamentally important.

Menage admitted that she was unable to ascertain whether the trauma of the intervention was totally due to the intervention itself, or whether there was a pre-existing element of PTSD due to a previous experience. This dilemma was addressed in a questionnaire survey of 289 women in London (Ayers and Pickering, 2001). The existence and level of PTSD was measured at thirty-six weeks' gestation and at six weeks and six months postnatally. During pregnancy eighteen women (8.1 per cent) were found to have PTSD and were excluded from subsequent data analysis. Seven new cases of PTSD were identified at six weeks, suggesting that the experience of birth may be a trigger factor for PTSD. These quantitative studies have been criticised (Moyzakitis, 2004) on the grounds that the instruments used had been designed for use following war and other large-scale conflicts involving men predominantly. Moyzakitis went on to identify the vulnerable women and the interventions in labour which could result in the new mother feeling traumatised. Such trauma may be doubly significant, because it not only affects the woman's emotional well-being, but also damages family relationships (Beech, 1998/9).

Although the significance of the traumatised new mother appears clear, research into her care is less so. 'Debriefing' has been widely welcomed as the solution to a number of postnatal problems (Steele and Beadle, 2003); its precise nature and aims, though, remain obscure. The role of the midwife has been demonstrated in reducing postnatal depression (Lavender and Walkinshaw, 1998; Small *et al.*, 2000), but these interventions do not yet appear to have been applied to women with PTSD (Joseph and Bailham, 2004).

Summary

It is apparent that, even in childbearing situations where the baby is born alive and well, there may still exist an element of regret. The mother may feel the loss of the fantasy baby to whom she did not give birth, of the baby of the 'right' gender who was not born or of the hoped-for birth experience which did not happen. These losses require the mother to grieve and may assume the proportions of a bereavement. It may be difficult for others to understand why a mother with an apparently ideal, or at least satisfactory, outcome has her moments or periods of sorrow. She may find it hard to acknowledge, even to herself. This mother may need our help to articulate and come to terms with her loss in the same way as any loss is eventually resolved.

In the care of mothers who are experiencing the birth of a healthy child, we should bear in mind the significance of loss. Grief is 'the other side of the coin' of the loving relationship which develops during pregnancy. Because this relationship is with an idealised fantasy baby and includes a range of other expectations, in the postnatal period she may need to grieve for not having fulfilled her fantasies and achieved her expectations.

3 Researching childbearing loss
Problems, dangers and opportunities

Certain essential questions, about the value of research and the use to which research-based knowledge is put, need to be asked. It is with these crucial questions that this chapter begins. Because researching perinatal grief carries certain inherent problems, I look at these next. Having already considered our use of research, I then look at its misuse; to do this I focus on examples of research becoming dogma, which we find in areas relating to grief and which raise fundamental issues. Finally, I look at how we may avoid such rigidity, by focusing on the design of my own study (Mander, 1992a), identifying a relevant research framework and highlighting outstanding research needs.

Do we need research?

As with any aspect of research, a question begins the process. Here, as I asked the midwives in my study, I ask: 'How do we know how to care for the grieving mother?' Many informants told me of the importance of experience, drawing on examples of their own childbearing and their occupational experience (Mander, 1992b). These midwives also recounted the limited contribution of formal methods of learning, such as lectures, refresher courses and reading nursing or midwifery journals. While recognising the importance of continuing education to knowledgeable and effective care, the crucial precursor is a questioning attitude to existing and proposed practices. This issue may be taken a stage further by suggesting that it is our *duty* to question established practice (Hicks, 1996). Their responses to my enquiry indicate the variable preparedness of midwives to question their practice:

IZZY: I always do my utmost to care as best I can. Care is really quite well done. I have never had any negative feedback. Really, I've not had very much contact afterwards at all.

GAY: I haven't had any training at all to help me to look after these mothers. . . . I think that the care that we give is quite reasonable. We give the mothers support and help and advice.

ANNIE: My ideas are my ideas. I don't know whether they are necessarily correct.

GINNIE: I often feel frustrated that I don't know what more I can do for them.
NELLIE: We try our best to give them as much time to talk to us as possible. But I feel that really that isn't as good as we should be doing.

As the comments by Ginnie and Nellie show, a questioning attitude may manifest itself when contemplating day-to-day practice. This may be supported by critical reading, the appropriate use of relevant research findings and, possibly, undertaking research. The reality of research implementation was noted by the Health Committee, who observed the lack of a research base for maternity care (House of Commons, 1992): 'Too many fashionable interventions . . . have been introduced without evaluation either of cost–benefit ratios or the reactions of women who undergo them.' Has our care of the grieving mother been based on 'fashionable interventions'? Our use of certain forms of treatment may constitute an unplanned, uncontrolled and unrecognised experiment. It is necessary to closely examine our care of the grieving mother and the knowledge on which it is based.

The development of research into perinatal grief

The knowledge-base which we use to care for the grieving mother originated with Sigmund Freud (1959 [1917]), who likened grief to a 'painful wound'. This helped dispense with the Judaeo-Christian view of grief, which regarded it as an unnecessary and unhelpful luxury; mourners were urged to avoid fruitless and unavailing grief. Freud, whose ideas were clinically derived, moved thinking in the direction of therapeutic support of bereaved people.

The first to systematically observe grief was Lindemann (1944). His, admittedly opportunistic, study sampled 101 of the people affected by the disastrous Cocoanut Grove night club fire. While not undervaluing his work, the narrow view which he took has been criticised. To describe grief, he should have taken into account or made allowance for the complex relationships between the bereaved and the deceased. Lindemann's tunnel vision serves as a reminder to avoid assumptions about others' grief based on personal value systems.

Founded on studies of the effects of separation on young institutionalised children, Bowlby's ideas moved grieving theory forward, by suggesting fundamental links between attachment and grief (1990). He hypothesised that, without loving attachment, there can be no loss. Thus, grief is the price that we as human beings pay for the joy of loving: often known as 'the cost of commitment'.

The close and powerful links between Bowlby's ideas and those of Parkes (1996) are clearly apparent, although their research populations were at opposite extremes of the age range. Parkes researched the grief of widows, as have many others. Unlike previous researchers, Parkes was able to demonstrate the contribution of the wider social community by demonstrating the value of relatively 'low-tech' interventions, such as bereavement counselling.

The significance of counselling is enhanced by his observation of the widespread and harmful effects of the stigma of loss, which may result in social deprivation.

Parkes's ideas were utilised by Forrest and colleagues (1982) when they researched support and counselling after perinatal bereavement. They, like Parkes, emphasise the long-term counselling of the family, compared with the supportive midwifery interventions at the birth and death. In an experimental design involving fifty mothers of babies who had died perinatally, half of the mothers received 'ideal' supported care, while the 'contrast' group received care of the usual variable standard.

The supported group were encouraged to see, hold and name their dead baby. The baby was photographed. The mother chose, whenever possible, where she was cared for and her transfer home was unhurried. Bereavement counselling was offered to both parents within two days of their loss. While the counselled mothers recovered from their grief more quickly than the contrast group, by the fourteen-month assessment there was no significant difference between the two groups. These findings are largely reassuring, though it may be that the intervention served only to 'hurry' the grief of the supported group. It is necessary to wonder, apart from the pain being longer lasting, whether marginally longer grief automatically reflects less effective grief. The significance of the high drop-out rate from the supported group is another cause for concern (see Chapter 6).

Recent research into perinatal grief reactions has suggested that the picture of how grief progresses is even less clear than was previously assumed. An authoritative study by Lin and Lasker (1996) suggests that the onset and progress of perinatal grief are affected by a range of personal factors. The sample included 163 women, and 56 of their partners, who were bereaved through miscarriage, stillbirth or neonatal death. As with most grief research, the attrition rate was high and only 122 parents (55.7 per cent) completed all three interviews. The analysis of these parents' grief scores over the two years following their loss showed four patterns of grieving:

1   In 41.0 per cent of parents there was a steady decline in the grief scores. This was described as a 'normal' pattern and was associated with being the mother and with a subsequent successful pregnancy.

2   In 13.1 per cent of parents the grief scores increased and this group was referred to as the 'reversed' grief group. In this group there was a low proportion of previous pregnancy losses and a high proportion of subsequent pregnancy losses.

3   The 'delayed' resolution group comprised 17.2 per cent of the parents. At the first interview they had relatively low scores but by the second, the grief score was highest. This group had the highest proportion of late pregnancy losses and of previous losses.

4   The fourth group, the 'low' unchanged group, showed grief scores which remained steady and low throughout the study and consisted of 28.7 per

cent of the parents. This group comprised a larger proportion of fathers and parents who had a larger proportion of children when the loss happened.

This study reminds us of the long-term nature of grief and the many factors which affect it.

In the course of their study of post traumatic stress disorder (PTSD) after giving birth to a stillborn baby, Hughes and colleagues' findings contradict the currently accepted wisdom (2002). These researchers found that, in a subsequent pregnancy, women who had seen and held their dead baby were more likely to be depressed, anxious and suffering from symptoms of PTSD than women who had done neither. User-group representatives have been appropriately critical of this study (Kohner, 2002). Because the focus of this study was on the care provided, more attention will be given to it in Chapter 5.

Issues arising out of previous research

The gestation or age at which the baby is lost has received much research attention (Singg, 2003: 882). This may be due to either the traditional assumption of the less-known being less grieved or to our increasing understanding of how the emotional relationship develops during pregnancy (see Chapter 2). Contrary to traditional assumptions, parents of newborns who die have been found to grieve more successfully than other bereaved parents (Murray and Callan, 1988). On the other hand, an authoritative review suggests that there are no significant differences between the grief of women losing their babies through miscarriage, stillbirth or neonatal death (Carter, 2003). Despite such research, the grief of the mother who miscarries is still denigrated. An example is the diktat by Bourne and Lewis (1991) that 'people should not be pushed into magnifying miscarriage'. Rather than magnifying or denigrating any mother's grief, I venture to suggest that we should accept her loss for what it means to her.

The effects on family relationships have attracted research attention, focusing mainly on differences in grieving between mother and father and any ensuing disharmony (Samuelsson *et al.*, 2001). The father's experience of loss is not yet well understood. This is partly due to the traditional focus on the mother's experience. It is also due in no small part to the difficulty of recruiting and collecting data from the father, as found in the study by Fiona Murphy (1998). I consider the implications for fathers and couples in Chapter 7.

The serious deficit in research-based knowledge into the effects of childbearing loss on siblings is well recognised (Robinson and Mahon, 1997). In Chapter 7 I examine the research by Dyregrov (1991) on perinatal sibling loss. This has helped to fill the void, although a retrospective approach, uncertainty about whether it was therapy or research and reliance on mothers' accounts of their children's loss limit the value of his work.

By predicting and measuring grief, attempts have been made to identify those most at risk of disordered grieving and to evaluate helpful interventions. Predictors were sought among 130 parents who had experienced perinatal loss by using a self-administered questionnaire (Murray and Callan, 1988). This obtained, as well as demographic data, features of the loss, levels of professional support and psychological well-being. Like others before them, these researchers found that better-supported parents grieved more healthily, endorsing our usual assumption that those who are less supported face worse outcomes. These researchers, though, made the mistake of focusing on professional interventions and not taking account of the grieving parents' social support system. It may be that the holistic view ordinarily adopted by nurses and midwives makes them ideally suited to fill this gap in our knowledge.

Criticisms of care inevitably arise when bereaved mothers are asked to recount their experiences. For all mothers we must take these criticisms seriously, although we may wonder, for those interviewed while still actively grieving, whether this may be a way of deciding whom to blame. In her retrospective study of fifteen mothers who had experienced perinatal loss, Hermione Lovell and colleagues (1986) found that mothers sensed the limited time staff were able or willing to spend with them. She also found that the community midwives' visits were variably appreciated. The medical checks six weeks postnatally were under-utilised, being merely physical in their orientation. This observation may be related to a phenomenon identified in a study of women who had experienced childbearing loss (Moulder, 1998). This is that the difficulty staff feel in coping with death may prevent them from supporting the mother. The limited social support offered to the grieving mother by the so-called community has also been identified (Mander, 1996).

In my study many of the relinquishing mothers were critical of certain aspects of their care; I have termed these experiences 'cock-ups'. Like other mothers, Jessica had been told not to have any contact with her baby; unfortunately this message was not communicated to all the staff caring for her:

JESSICA: Just after the baby was born I was in a room with all the other mothers. He was in my arms for about an hour. There was some kind of mix-up, because when my parents came in at night he had been brought out to me again. By that time I had been put in a side room by myself. I had him that night and I was quite happy with myself. The next day the nurses said that was it! I couldn't have any more contact! Then one of the midwives said to me 'That bond hasn't got to be there. You can't bond. You can't see him any more.'

As well as raising issues about the bonding doctrine (please see Chapter 2), this example shows that, when communication between staff breaks down, the mother is left feeling confused and insecure.

Midwifery research has been shown, despite its significance mentioned already, to be undervalued by midwives themselves (Hicks, 1992). In a small and questionably ethical study, Hicks shows that midwives rate a research report significantly more highly if they believe it to be written by a medical practitioner rather than a midwife. Hicks concludes that research is not perceived as being essential to midwifery, but she omits to recognise the prevailing value system.

Methodological issues

There are certain issues which are particularly important in the planning and utilisation of research into childbearing loss. One of these is its quality, because it has been argued that 'careless research is as immoral as careless surgery' (Davis, 1983). Although terms like 'bad' research are bandied about, they mean little more than 'research methods which I have not used and don't understand'. Such deprecatory terms may be used by 'hard-edged' researchers to describe qualitative approaches, and I suspect that their insecurity with unfamiliar methods lies at the root of the difficulty. It may be that truly immoral research is that which is done at some cost to the respondents and to the funding body, but which is never reported or disseminated to practitioners (Mander, 1995a).

The **design** of many grief research projects is criticised for using a retrospective approach, inevitably relying on recall. A grief-stricken memory is likely to distort the data and result in bias. The longitudinal prospective study is a valuable alternative, which may provide accurate current data, but unfortunately a time lapse may be necessary to allow the bereaved mother to recover from the worst pain of her grief (Leon, 1990: 189).

The **sample** needs to be selected to minimise risks to subjects, such as causing pain or impairing grieving. As always, the sample size should to be the smallest number possible consistent with being suitably representative.

The **response rate** indicates the acceptability and importance which the members of the population attach to the research. A low response rate raises questions of whether those who did not respond differ significantly from those who did (Murphy-Black, 2000). In grief research it is to be expected that the response rate will be low compared with other topics. Obviously, this reflects only those studies which actually state the response rate as this information is all too often omitted. It is necessary to remember the risk of 'attenuation' of the sample, which in quantitative research reduces the likelihood of statistically significant findings.

The **representativeness** of the sample may be hampered by the nature of the study, as those who agree to be involved may be grieving atypically. Perhaps it is only those whose grief is progressing smoothly who agree to participate, or, alternatively, those who need more help hope to get it through involvement in research?

The identification of a suitable sample is addressed by Worden (2003), who discusses the diverse social groupings and distances which a researcher may need to cover. The nature of grief requires that the sample must be, like Lindemann's (see page 21), an opportunistic or convenience sample, thus reducing the researcher's control over the study. Research into childbearing loss may be particularly problematical because of the difficulty of finding a suitable sample when so many potentially different forms of loss are included.

Researching grief brings certain unique or particular problems. Especially likely is the Hawthorne effect, when the subject changes their behaviour because of their involvement in research. Such a change clearly invalidates the data.

Worden (2003) focuses on problems associated with measuring grief by using health as an indicator. Proxy measures may be used, as these may be more accessible than health data. Examples include medication, GP contacts or hospital admission. Symptoms are, thus, inappropriately regarded as manifestations of grief, whereas these 'health behaviours' may be even more culture-bound and socially determined than grief itself. Further, treatment may be more closely related to help-seeking variables than to the person's degree of disturbance. It may be that medication is the least reliable proxy for grief, as the values of the prescriber also complicate the picture.

The hazards of grief research make themselves abundantly clear in the project undertaken by DiMarco and her colleagues in the USA (2001). A largely quantitative, retrospective two-group design was employed to evaluate the benefits of support group involvement. The sampling frame was the mailing list for a 'perinatal loss support newsletter' (2001: 136). This sampling frame implies that both groups are already receiving some support, with the potential to reduce differences. The two comparison groups comprised parents who did or chose not to attend the support group, introducing an element of bias. The response rate was low at 32 per cent (128 individuals out of 400 approached) in spite of two follow-up mailings. The response from fathers was particularly poor, at approximately one-third of the number of mothers responding. These problems of accessing and retaining a suitable sample are familiar to grief researchers.

The danger of dogma

We have considered already the reasons why research-based knowledge is crucial to inform our care of the grieving mother and the benefits which accrue. Because examples arise in our care, it is necessary to turn our minds to the potential for less beneficial effects of research. By this, I mean research having been elevated to dogma which, by definition, one questions at one's peril.

The first example of research being used to justify dogma is found in what has become known as the bonding doctrine, resulting in mothers being harassed when they are least able to question their care. Taking a historical perspective, a series of child-care gurus whose ideas have initially required adherence have subsequently been challenged and eventually rejected. Unlike the instantaneous, cataclysmic, all-or-nothing 'gluing', as it is all too often presented, the mother–baby relationship grows gradually, through learning to know and coming to understand each other. There are clearly certain factors which hinder this relationship from developing, just as there are others which facilitate it.

Another example of research being elevated to dogma is more closely related to our present topic. Bourne and Lewis (1991) warn us of the danger that certain forms of care may be applied universally as a panacea to 'solve' the mother's grief. Their examples include the formerly widespread recommendation 'have another' (see Chapter 13). They suggest that many of our interventions may be effective only in the short term. Their scorn at recommendations for caring for the mother who miscarries ignores research emphasising the grief of miscarriage (SPCERH, 2003) and reminds us of the shaky statistical foundation on which our current care of the mother experiencing perinatal loss is built (Leon, 1990).

Another example of potentially dangerous dogma is found in the research by Hughes and colleagues (2002), which may serve to highlight the possibly damaging effect of what they term the 'current fashion' for the mother having contact with her dead baby. These researchers argue that a practice which may have begun life as 'sensitive care' only 'traumatises a woman who is already intensely distressed and physically exhausted' (2002: 117).

A third way in which dogma becomes significant in the context of research into childbearing loss is in the design of the research. The views of those who are responsible for approving access for research, the 'gatekeepers', encounter difficulty understanding research which incorporates ideas or methods with which they are not familiar. For this reason they may be wary of approving research proposals which do not comply with their attitudes to 'patients' or with their positivistic views of research. In my study, her limited view of the role of the midwife prevented one social worker from co-operating (Mander, 1992c). Another's conviction that grief was a short-term phenomenon had a similar effect. Limited understanding of grieving also became apparent in correspondence with research ethics committees (RECs). Criticisms of the research method related to the flexible nature of my data collection, being equated with 'sociological-type' and, hence, 'bad' research.

For these reasons, I propose that we as carers read research critically, use it questioningly and undertake appropriately designed studies, rather than being vulnerable to the whims of medical or even psychological fashion.

A study of loss

As I became aware of the demise of the 'rugger pass' approach to the care of the mother grieving perinatal death, I sought to learn whether more enlightened approaches are also being applied to the care of the mother relinquishing her baby for adoption. I describe here the design of a study which I undertook to investigate this issue; methodological issues relating to the avoidance of dogma in research design become evident.

The research approach

The lack of previous research on midwives' care of the relinquishing mother and its innately sensitive nature led me to choose a qualitative research approach with some quantitative elements. Qualitative research seeks to understand the event from the perspective of the person experiencing it – the 'emic' approach (Kaye, 1994). A holistic picture of the phenomenon emerges, demonstrating the interrelatedness and interdependence of differing facets of the event (Silverman and Klass, 1996).

Although some argue that this approach is 'soft' and 'unscientific', this is probably a strength in the present context, because the qualitative approach is well suited to the descriptive focus which was used to understand the subjective viewpoint of the mother and her interpretation of her relinquishment.

The advantages of large-scale studies of the effects of grief may be compared with smaller-scale in-depth research (Stroebe and Stroebe, 1987). The epidemiological data collected in the former serve a different purpose from the 'fine-grained' details on matters such as coping strategies obtained in the latter. Thus, the researcher chooses between statistical significance and in-depth insight into the phenomenon, depending on the research questions.

I included both qualitative and quantitative elements to constitute triangulation at the level of the research design (Denzin and Lincoln, 2000), to further increase the rigour of the data.

The research questions

On the basis of the literature available and personal experience six research questions emerged:

1   What is the experience of the mother relinquishing her baby?
2   To what extent are the experiences of relinquishing mothers in the UK similar to those of mothers in other countries?
3   How, in the midwife's view, does the care she gives to a relinquishing mother differ from that provided for another mother without a baby?
4   How are decisions made regarding the midwife's care of the relinquishing mother?
5   What knowledge is involved in making these decisions?
6   How is this knowledge acquired?

The method

I planned the fieldwork in three phases, examining the viewpoints of those involved. These were, first, previous relinquishing mothers (who had relinquished a baby in the past), second, experienced midwives and, third, current relinquishing mothers (planning relinquishment).

- **Phase 1** – to assess the relevance of other countries' literature on long-term feelings about relinquishment by interviewing mothers who had previously relinquished a baby.
- **Phase 2** – to explore the care provided by the midwife, with particular reference to whether her care of a relinquishing mother differs from that provided for another mother without a baby. Interviews would be held with a sample of experienced midwives.
- **Phase 3** – to observe and then describe the experience of the relinquishing mother using a prospective, longitudinal technique. Interviews with a small group of mothers would focus on the experience of giving birth while at the same time making the decision to relinquish her baby. The extent to which her midwifery care had affected the experience would be sought. An interview would be held in the woman's home shortly after the birth and a similar interview would be held some months later to ascertain whether her impressions of her care had developed in any way.

Obtaining permission for research access

Gaining access to the research site involved obtaining ethical approval (for phase 3) and permission from midwife managers. Because it had been necessary to recruit previous relinquishing mothers from a wide area, I decided to recruit midwives from a similar area. My approaches elicited enthusiastic, sympathetic and helpful support and the managers gave permission for me to seek the midwives' participation. Midwives were given permission to be interviewed in their on-duty time at their work place, if they wished.

Access to a suitable sample of relinquishing mothers for phase 1 was unproblematic after making contact with birth parents' groups, whose organisers and members were keen to participate (Mander, 1992c). The relinquishing mothers comprised a volunteer sample. The midwives were randomly selected from off-duty lists. Ethical approval and access for phase 3 presented major difficulties. Eventually a case-study approach was utilised for the one mother I was able to recruit (Mander, 1992d).

The instrument and personal implications

I used a semi-structured interview format, allowing the informant to control the topics, although my introduction reiterated my area of interest, which I had explained during the initial contact. My frequently updated interview schedule comprised a list of questions, in addition to which I encouraged the mothers to introduce relevant issues. My questions were based on the literature, my occupational and other experience and, in later interviews, issues raised by earlier informants. The interviews were tape-recorded with the informant's permission.

An essential feature of this form of fieldwork is the way in which I, the researcher, present and use my personality during the interview. This applies to such an extent that my personality constitutes part of the research instrument, by interacting with the data. This contrasts with the usual requirement for the researcher to be a neutral 'non-person' to avoid bias.

The researcher must be conscious of any intuitive or personal reactions to the informant or her information. Examples would be revulsion when 'Francesca' recounted the behaviour of her peers in an alien subculture, or sorrow at 'Quelia's' pathetically limited outlook on life, or overwhelming feelings of identification due to a common early post-war working-class background with 'Barbara' and 'Debra'. Feelings of identification or a shared orientation with the informant may or may not be helpful. Such commonalities may be reasons for not participating. Clearly, assumptions of empathy on the part of the researcher may not help the research. By being aware of such reactions we are able to take account of them in both the fieldwork and the analysis of the data.

For the researcher, emotional discomfort may follow such personal involvement (Mander, 1999a). One of the RECs questioned how I would cope with the emotional impact of undertaking a study involving such deep powerful feelings. This may be through a supporting team of researchers who are able to share problems. For this small study, however, this was not possible and I relied on domestic, collegial and social support.

The emotional toll which research takes is particularly significant in qualitative studies, where personal involvement with the work, if not the informants, is crucial. This aspect is only now beginning to be addressed and the 'cost of involvement' in research into sensitive topics is being brought out into the open (Mander, 2000).

Completion of the fieldwork and data analysis

Field notes captured my immediate impressions and reactions to the informant and her data. I incorporated the themes into subsequent interviews. After I had listened to the recording of the interview, it was transcribed on to disk. I checked the hard copy with the taped interview, to correct errors and colloquial and technical terms.

By the time I had interviewed twenty-three previous relinquishing mothers and forty midwives, no new conceptual categories were emerging and the data had become saturated. Thus, no more interviews were required.

Data analysis began during the fieldwork using comparative analysis, in which I compared newly acquired with existing data, to determine how they related to each other. Thus, theory was constantly developing, being revised and determining the direction of future fieldwork.

In exploring the experience of relinquishment and the provision of midwifery care, I sought insights to illuminate the essential aspects of that care. This exploration was completed after each phase of the fieldwork by using analytic description, involving active inspection of the transcripts, in an attempt to identify novel categories to describe the phenomenon. This method of analysis ensured that all of the essential findings had been explained (Denzin and Lincoln, 2000).

The hard copy was coded using categories which seemed appropriate from my reading of and listening to the interviews. There were about 200 categories for the relinquishing mothers and a similar number for the midwives. Some of the categories were common to both groups, but there were many which were relevant only to one group of informants, such as midwives' accounts of learning about grieving. These codes were transferred on to disk by the typist and this permitted categorised statements to be extracted from the disk copy and reformed into about twenty categories, each of which focused on one area. Examination of each of these categories, including a count, provided me with a complete impression of the varying aspects, including the salience, of that topic (Fielding and Lee, 1991).

Terminology

Anonymity and confidentiality are vital to these informants, so throughout I used fictitious names. Names ending with 'y' or 'e' (Amy, Betty, Annie, Bessie . . .) denote midwives, whereas relinquishing mothers have been given names ending with 'a' (Anthea, Barbara, etc.). Other potentially identifying material was altered.

The opportunities: outstanding research needs

There are many areas relating to childbearing loss in need of research attention.

Maternity care for the grieving mother

We have considered already in this chapter the dangers of under-researched interventions being applied dogmatically. While Forrest *et al.* (1982) looked at the effects of interventions to assist grieving, their research design incorporated a 'package'; the constituent parts were not clearly distinguishable, leaving concerns about which parts were effective. If we are to establish the value of interventions and avoid dogma, it is necessary for us to learn more about how mothers perceive their care. An example would be the care of the mother's breasts and whether she lactates (see Chapter 5).

The organisation of the care of the grieving mother deserves attention, in that we should find out whether a 'team approach' comprising highly trained and experienced specialists is more acceptable to the mother than the usual pattern of care (Primeau and Lamb, 1995).

Midwives are accustomed to teaching mothers and others about various aspects of childbearing, but little is known about what is taught to mothers about grief or whether that teaching is effective. It is necessary for us to find out what education is provided and whether the mother and others perceive it as helpful (see Chapter 5).

The care of the mother in the community

The midwives in my study were uniformly convinced of the value of the mother being transferred home promptly:

HILARY: She should have as short a stay in hospital as possible. In hospital she may be forced to bottle up her emotions. Hospitals are really very busy places, much too busy to allow her to grieve. She should go home to be with her own people and have the chance to be in her own environment.

This widespread assumption contrasts with the observations by Alice Lovell (1984, 1997) and Rajan (1994), who identified the mother's perception of being despatched home over-hastily and not for her benefit, but because the staff in the maternity unit had difficulty coping with her presence (see Chapter 5). The decision about the mother's transfer home, particularly who makes it, what influences it and how it relates to education about grieving, deserves closer attention.

The return home may not be the panacea which mothers and midwives anticipate. The grieving mother found that her friends and family had other preoccupations which limited the support available. If we continue to transfer the grieving mother home quickly, we should at least know the environment to which she is returning and how it compares with the maternity unit.

Although they were convinced that the mother would find good support when she returned home, the midwives in my study were uncertain about the same people as visitors in the maternity unit:

QUEENY: The patient is in control of who comes to see her. If she decides she only wants to see her husband today, then that is who she sees. If there is too much of a crowd we may say something.

While this may reflect a common area of conflict, the implications for the grieving mother are particularly serious. We should give attention to the discrepancy between family visiting in the maternity unit needing supervision and assuming the family at home are supportive. Although the midwives, like Queeny, were happy for the mother to decide who visited, I was unable to find out what help, if any, the mother was given in making and implementing this decision.

Mothers' evaluations of community midwives' home visits vary hugely (Lovell *et al.*, 1986). The significance of this opportunity to provide continuing education and support for the grieving mother should not be underestimated, but existing reports suggest that it is not well utilised (see Chapter 5). The factors affecting the benefits of these visits need attention.

Staff issues

As recognised in Chapters 10 and 11, maternity staff have difficulty coping with death, and this may affect their care of the mother. Various strategies have been and are being used to support staff in coping with death, ranging from 'We're off to the pub' to formal psychologist-led sessions. In view of the serious implications of staff support for all concerned, information is needed on how best it may be organised.

Other issues

The problems of the mother with a **known stillbirth** (see Chapter 4) and who is aware of carrying a dead baby are unique. Her care is influenced by the way in which her grief progresses before her baby is born, but little is currently known about her grieving. To care for this mother optimally, we need a more complete picture of how her grief progresses.

As I show in Chapter 12, midwives are generally confident to recommend mothers to seek help from **self-help groups**. The basis of this confidence is unclear and the benefits of these groups deserve research (Watson, 1993).

Mothers belonging to **ethnic minority groups** are generally neglected by researchers. Loss is one example of the lack of research relating to minority groups and demonstrates the ethnocentricity of UK health care (Douglas, 1992). If we are to care appropriately for mothers of different ethnic backgrounds, information about their interpretation of their loss is urgently needed.

Summary

In this chapter I have considered the significance of research in caring for the grieving mother. I have shown its importance for those who provide care and, indirectly, for the mother herself. After suggesting that research may occasionally be used inappropriately, I have shown how I used a suitably flexible research approach. Finally, I have identified some aspects of loss in childbearing which need research attention.

4 Features of loss in childbearing

There are certain situations, other than those which come easily to mind, when a mother faces grief. I have already considered the concept of grief in uncomplicated, healthy childbearing in Chapter 2. I now consider losses which engender more profound and enduring grief. In this chapter I focus, first, on those features of loss in childbearing which prolong or inhibit grieving. Second, I contemplate certain examples of loss which may present special difficulty.

Unique features of loss which may adversely affect grieving

To examine the unique features, I utilise Davidson's theoretical framework which was based on interviews with fifteen families with experience of perinatal death (1977). He identified certain aspects of loss which engendered conflict and confusion and, thus, impeded healthy grieving.

Confirming perceptually who died

Due to certain unique factors, the fact of the loss of her baby is hard to accept, or may even be resisted, by the mother. Lewis and Bourne (1989) attribute her reaction to the uncertain and bewildering circumstances in which she 'half knows' her baby, but has never seen her. These writers liken her predicament to that following 'missing, presumed dead' verdicts.

Unreality – Ordinarily, when someone dies after the usual life-span, those who are left have a variety of tangible and intangible memories. If there is loss in childbearing, these memories don't exist. The mother may have memories of her baby's movements before the birth or she may recall imaginary 'conversations', perhaps willing her baby to quieten down to sleep or pleading with her to be born to end a seemingly interminable pregnancy. The baby's father has even less by which to remember her, perhaps only being kicked in the back at night.

The mother's lack of tangible **memories** leaves her wondering 'What am I grieving for?' She may recall a fleeting contact at birth, when she was in a less than ideal state to take everything in. But, as she is mourning a person who is unseen and unknown in the usual way, she finds that the reality of her loss is missing. If the mother's grieving is to proceed, she has to accept that her baby has been born and has been lost through death or in another way. This loss means, inevitably, that the baby will not return or be miraculously brought back. Acceptance of the reality of her loss may be assisted by rehearsing the events, either in her mind or with another person.

Just as the lack of memories makes grieving difficult, the lack of a **focus for grief** may also make loss in childbearing unreal. The coffin and funeral have traditionally provided a short-term focus for grief and the grave has been a source of longer-term reminiscences. But recently ritual has been dispensed with and unmarked graves or cremation have deprived the mother of a focus for her grief.

The importance of such a focus impressed itself on me in the culture in which I grew up, where mourners return to the house of the dead person and either choose or are given something which belonged to her. It may be an item of clothing, a household object or even a houseplant. Although I initially found it macabre, I soon learned that this object gives the mourner something concrete on which to focus their grief.

Loss of self – The lack of tangible mementoes of a lost baby lends greater significance to those intangible, unseen and usually unspoken fantasies which only the person experiencing them understands. Having been biologically created by her parents, the baby has not only their genetic make-up; she also has invested in her their hopes, dreams and aspirations. It may be that parents commit themselves in their baby, in the hope that she will develop to gratify their unfulfilled wishes and unachieved ambitions. Thus, she represents not only a biological, but also a psychological, extension of her parents. These dreams and aspirations reflect only those characteristics of the mother which she most admires or loves in herself, hence the wish to pass them on. These narcissistic expectations for her child are dashed if the child is lost, leaving her to grieve not only for her child, but also for some part of herself which may be indistinguishable from her child.

Untimeliness – A mother grieving the loss of her child represents an upset in the usual order of things, and exacerbates the confusion and loss of control which she feels. These feelings may be aggravated by the mother's perception of herself and her child as a part of the ongoing tapestry of life, which has been brought to an abrupt end. Hence, for parents who regard their child as their 'stake in eternity' a fundamental threat has been posed to the continuity of life, adding a new and frightening significance to their own mortality. Elements of survivor guilt may leave the mother feeling 'It should have been me', further increasing her confusion.

Lack of contact – The mother, like others, may have mistakenly believed that love only develops when the baby is seen and known (Bowlby, 1990). Because they assume that little contact means no affection, it may be thought that no loving mother–child relationship exists. Hence, because she is not regarded as a 'proper' mother, both the mother and those nearby have difficulty accepting the mother's profound and enduring grief. In contrast to her expectations, the mother may be alarmed by the strength of her emotions, making her fear for her sanity. For the same reason, those near her denigrate her grief, and may encourage her to 'pull herself together'.

Getting emotional support

The non-involvement in childbearing of those who would ordinarily give support may, in turn, limit the help available in the event of loss.

Intimacy of loss – Because, in childbearing, the number of people who have any direct or intimate contact with the unborn baby is unlikely to be more than two, there is limited scope for community support. As mentioned already, those not intimately involved have difficulty comprehending the significance of the loss, causing them to make unintentionally hurtful 'Have another'-type comments. This difficulty has led to grieving parents being regarded as having no right to grieve; they become *illegitimate* mourners. Emotional support is soon withdrawn from those perceived as being undeserving of it. Those who are grieving quickly realise the futility of seeking help and, so, conceal their emotions, creating a 'conspiracy of silence' and aggravating feelings of the birth having been a 'non-event' (Rådestad *et al.*, 1996a).

Complexity of emotional processes – I have shown that the depth of grief experienced at this time may be hard for both the mother and those near to her to understand. This jeopardises her support. The complexity of her emotions may be similarly incomprehensible and damaging.

The mother is effectively attempting to say 'Hello' and 'Goodbye' simultaneously. During pregnancy, the focus is to prepare a suitable physical and emotional environment in which the new arrival may be nurtured. As the pregnancy advances the momentum of preparations increases, so that completing the necessary emotional 'about-turn', in the event of loss, is a major problem. In Chapter 13, I discuss the problems which women have been said to encounter if they conceive while mourning. The problems of the new mother mourning her baby are marginally less, as she must cease her optimistic preparations while grieving the end of the mother–child relationship (Lewis and Bourne, 1989).

Relative youth of parents – Women in their childbearing years are relatively young and are unlikely to be acquainted with grief. The mother will not, therefore, have had opportunities to develop coping strategies to help her through this experience of loss. Thus, her grief becomes a crisis for which, by definition, any previous coping strategies are inappropriate (Caplan, 1961). The ineffective coping strategies utilised by younger bereaved parents feature anger and outrage. While their older equivalents also grieve angrily, their anger is underpinned by fear of remaining childless as the mother's biological clock ticks inexorably on.

Appropriate emotional support – While emotional support may be forthcoming, the mother has difficulty identifying who is prepared to offer her sufficiently intensive and enduring support. I discuss family and carers support in Chapters 7 and 10 respectively.

Comparing her feelings with those of others

The non-comprehension of the mother's grief by those from whom she ordinarily takes her behavioural cues leaves her feeling unsupported.

Meaning of the pregnancy – The mother's perception of poor support causes her to feel alone and isolated in her grief. One of the factors which aggravate her loneliness is the uniqueness of the meaning which she attaches to her pregnancy. This is because, as mentioned already, when a child is conceived a variety of unique hopes, expectations and aspirations develop in those who are involved. If a baby is lost, these dreams are also lost and, in the same way as the dreams were unique, so is the grief following their loss, leaving her isolated in her grief (Lewis and Bourne, 1989).

Contrasting her own earlier expectations – The media and health care providers emphasise the ease and normality of childbearing (DeVries, 1996). This emphasis, together with the widespread silence surrounding perinatal loss, successfully shields us from the, relatively infrequent, tragic outcomes. So, if problems happen, events are shockingly different from expectations; the mother's confidence is shaken and her self-esteem plummets.

Similar assumptions which we make about the ease of childbearing result in an overwhelming focus on control, that is prevention, of fertility by contraception. When faced with involuntary infertility, the reality is a shocking contrast to our usual assumptions. The contrast between expectations and reality applies at a fundamental level to all aspects of 'reproductive failure'. Until problems are encountered, fertility is little more than an, occasionally inconvenient, basic human function. But when we find that the desired level of fertility is beyond our grasp, our human integrity is threatened.

Examples of loss in childbearing

In addition to these issues which apply generally, each of the more profound forms of loss carries unique features, some of which have been researched.

Stillbirth

As I have suggested already, this is a topic which is not discussed socially despite families having knowledge or experience of it. I realised this when I first entered midwifery and mothers told me that the shop always kept the new pram until after the birth – 'in case anything happens'. The possibility of stillbirth was recognised implicitly, together with an element of magical thinking to avoid tempting fate.

The existing research on this subject has focused on reactions to stillbirth, and care after the birth to help cope with those reactions. Probably for this reason, little attention has been given to the two significantly different forms of stillbirth, 'known' and 'unexpected', and their emotional implications.

Known stillbirth

Sometimes referred to as 'intra-uterine death' (IUD), the process of maceration of the baby's body may begin, depending on the length of time between her death and her birth.

The mother's grieving may be affected by how long she is aware of carrying her dead baby within her. It may be that the mother would be the first to note the cessation of fetal movements and realise its significance. This leads us to wonder whether this realisation assists grieving. While grieving may begin only when the baby separates from the mother at birth, it may be that the mother, beneficially, begins grieving while pregnant. She may at least experience shock and denial to begin her grieving prior to the birth or, alternatively, she may begin anticipatory grieving (see Chapter 8). In a small study, women who had noted the absence of fetal movements did not realise the significance of this observation (Moulder, 1998), so they were seriously disturbed when fetal demise was confirmed. Authoritative research evidence is needed to show how this woman's grief develops, if we are to offer her the most appropriate care.

Carrying a dead baby – The feeling of empty stillness which the mother senses within her symbolises the end of her relationship with her baby. No longer does her body house a person who is going to provide gratification, but she now comes to despise parts of her body that once provided recognition and pleasure.

I will never forget my sense of repugnance when I first learned that a mother with a known stillbirth was coming into the labour ward for a third attempt to induce her labour. I soon realised that her feelings of horror could only be worse, probably akin to the perception of being a 'living coffin' (Jolly, 1987). Profound disturbances in a mother's body image feature feelings of uncleanness, which may be associated with her sense of revulsion at retaining her dead baby. Forrest (1983) understates the fantasies of such mothers in her sample, describing them as 'unpleasant'. When they voiced concerns about how their babies were physically changing, they were accused of being 'morbid' or 'ghoulish'.

Inducing labour – Because of the physical changes in the baby, the likely emotional reaction and the risk of the mother developing a clotting disorder, induction of labour is usually recommended (Zorlu *et al.*, 1997). Traditionally, this induction has been begun speedily, although the labour tends to be prolonged. Now greater flexibility pertains about who decides whether and when the induction happens. Dyer (1992) encourages her to wait 'a day or two' for the induction after learning of her loss in order to reorientate herself.

Assuming that she will see her baby, the changes in the baby's body may affect the mother's decision about when to have labour induced. Delaying the induction may signify continuing denial, although this need not be an indication for early induction. The mother deciding the timing of the induction may be one way for her to assume control of an otherwise uncontrollable situation (see page 35). Midwives in my study encouraged this mother to assume control (Mander, 1992d):

OTTILY: [Induction] is an obstetrician's decision though, but I think that they move too fast sometimes and that may not be good for the woman; it may not be healthy for her. It seems to be a case of 'get it over and done with'. I think that this may be for the benefit of the staff – for us. One woman was asked to come in that same afternoon. She didn't come in and she actually turned up three days later. We had been in touch with her GP to check that there were no real problems and it seemed to be all right. She waited until she felt that she was ready. But the labour is usually induced as soon as the diagnosis of fetal death has been made. This is probably blocking the realisation of the death. When it is being explained to the woman she would probably be told about the medical risks such as . . . coagulation problems.

Denial – If the woman is still protecting herself from the unacceptable news, the staff may be unable to convince her of the reality of her baby's death. I learned this when I was a new midwife in an antenatal ward and a mother with hypertension was admitted near term. Our observations suggested that her baby was dead, but she insisted that this was not so because her baby was still moving. Despite being gently informed of the situation, her denial persisted. Days later, she agreed to have labour induced because her baby was due and her blood pressure remained high. She was devastated when her daughter was stillborn.

It is necessary to consider the effect which denial may have on others, such as family. It is not, however, only mothers who use denial as protection; a midwife informant recounted her experience of known stillbirth:

ANNIE: There is a moment at the birth when everyone who is present, the parents and the staff, see that the baby has been born and hope against hope that the baby is going to cry. I know that it's quite illogical, but you still hope. And it is not until that moment when we all realise that the baby really is dead, then we all finally realise it is so.

Unexpected stillbirth

The baby may die unexpectedly in labour or during the birth and result in what has been known as a 'fresh stillbirth'. This death has all the characteristics of sudden death, with the parents experiencing shock and fear, with little time for the mythical bargaining. This form of stillbirth may only be recognised when we are unable to resuscitate a previously healthy baby who was in a poor condition at birth. Ethical questions arise when deciding how long to continue resuscitation attempts.

The unexpectedness of this form of loss presents a major challenge to the staff as well as the mother. Staff may question the reliability of their own observations which led to confidence in the baby's condition. They may find that those aspects of care which are ordinarily second nature, such as communication and information-giving, become unbearably difficult. In my experience, the mother's need for information and support may be overlooked while staff continue resuscitation attempts and prepare to face the prospect of a healthy fetus becoming a stillbirth or neonatal death.

Reactions after the birth

The depth of mothers' reactions to stillbirth has been demonstrated in the small number of studies focusing on this challenging time. Hsu and colleagues used an interpretive ethnographic approach to focus on the woman's interaction over the two-year period after the stillbirth (2002).

These researchers' most notable finding is the mother's universal expression of guilt at 'having caused' the death of the baby (2002: 391). The mother's coping strategies addressed, first, the meaning of the baby's death and her attempts to transform it into a less negative experience. Second, the mother sought to ameliorate her guilt by compensating for causing the baby's death. Third, a further way of reducing her feelings of guilt was by planning future pregnancies. The fourth and final coping strategy sought to address the social relationships damaged by the loss of the baby. Although this study was undertaken in Taiwan, these coping strategies are likely to be relevant to Western women.

The relevance of these coping strategies in the West is clearly endorsed by the work of Turton and colleagues (2001). These researchers collected data in the third trimester of the subsequent pregnancy. The data related to demographic variables, depression, anxiety and post traumatic stress disorder (PTSD). In the same way as Dyson and While (1998) identified the enduring nature of perinatal grief, Turton *et al.* demonstrated the heavy psychological burden which the woman bereaved by stillbirth carries with her. This burden was found by an Australian study to take the form of serious mental health problems, which could be either acute or chronic (Boyle, 1997). At two months after the death of the baby one-third of mothers exhibited anxiety and one-fifth depression. Although these rates fell markedly by the eighth month, thereafter the rates remained constant. The result was that, at 2.5 years anxiety rates (14 per cent) and depression rates (7 per cent) were significantly higher than those found in equivalent mothers whose babies had survived. Boyle and her colleagues relate their findings to the vulnerability of the women in their sample. This vulnerability takes the form of chronically poor social support being acutely exacerbated by the stressful experience of the loss of a baby. These negative effects do not appear to have been 'buffered' by the presence of existing children, as may sometimes be assumed.

The operation of support by professionals in the event of perinatal loss was addressed in a study in England (Moulder, 1998). This largely qualitative study identified the variability of the psychosocial support offered and, reciprocally, its variable acceptability and uptake. The effectiveness of professional support was related by the women to the nature of the relationship, how well established the relationship was at the time of the loss and its likely duration. The latter point meant that, although general practitioners might not be the preferred 'significant professional' (1998: 144), the fact that the relationship was not time limited, like that with the midwife, made it more easily acceptable.

Accidental loss in early pregnancy: miscarriage

A pregnancy may be accidentally lost before becoming viable which, in the UK, is set at 24 weeks' gestation. This loss may take one of a number of forms, including spontaneous abortion and ectopic pregnancy. Although the circumstances of the loss may differ, the word 'miscarriage' is widely used to include these various forms of loss (SPCERH, 2003). The term 'silent miscarriage' is a good example of a more sympathetic term which has been introduced to replace 'missed abortion'.

A common event

Although the loss of 'biological' pregnancies may be much higher (Lovell, 1997), clinically recognised miscarriages are estimated to occur in at least 10 to 20 per cent of all pregnancies (SPCERH, 2003). The frequency of miscarriage leads some to regard it as a 'normal' event. This information may be used to 'comfort' the woman who has experienced a miscarriage, by telling her that it is 'nature's way' of preventing the birth of a baby with disabilities. Such denigration of the experience may eventually lead to the baby being described as products of conception or 'POC' (Forna and Gülmezoglu, 2004).

Grieving miscarriage

Our traditional disregard of miscarriage may be attributable to, first, the non-visibility and resulting non-recognition of the pregnancy. Second, 'quickening' has in the past been assumed to be highly significant in the development of both the fetus and the mother–baby relationship, rendering early pregnancy loss less meaningful. Third, disregard of miscarriage has been made worse by our limited knowledge of the emotional processes of early pregnancy, which may include the assumption that shorter gestation carries less emotional investment. There is evidence to suggest that the emotional changes which assist the adjustment to parenthood may begin prior to conception (Rubin, 1967) and, in a large and authoritative study, it was found that there are no significant differences between the grief responses of women losing their babies through miscarriage, stillbirth or neonatal death (Peppers and Knapp, 1980). Assumption of 'no grief' following miscarriage may be little more than an admission of ignorance, because it is unlikely a follow-up will assess how this mother does or does not recover. It may be that, by dismissing this mother's emotional response to miscarriage, we are denying her the opportunity to grieve healthily.

Research into grief following miscarriage originally focused on the psychiatric sequelae. The value of early work to measure the emotional consequences of miscarriage has been questioned on the grounds of non-use of a standardised assessment (Friedman and Gath, 1989). These researchers used well-validated instruments to assess the mental health of sixty-seven women four weeks after miscarriage. The data showed that thirty-two (48 per cent) mothers were psychiatric 'cases', a rate four times higher than among women generally. Depressive conditions predominated and correlated with previous miscarriage rather than childlessness. Many of the mothers showed features characteristic of grief and some had attempted self-harm.

The experience of miscarriage

In view of the tendency, mentioned already, to denigrate the significance of miscarriage, Bansen and Stevens (1992) undertook a qualitative study to describe the experience of early miscarriage. The sample of ten mothers who had miscarried two to five months earlier was gathered through referrals and informal networking. The mothers had all lost a desired first pregnancy.

These researchers found profound guilt, anger at their bodies and fear for future childbearing. Most significantly, this study showed that miscarriage is not necessarily the insignificant menstruation-like event which it is sometimes thought; several mothers focused on the severe pain and heavy bleeding which were serious enough to engender fear of dying. The mother's grief was long-lasting; resolution may have been impeded by the sudden onset of the miscarriage, precluding any opportunities for anticipatory grieving. Social support was unforthcoming, which was compounded by unhelpful comments denigrating the loss. Regarding her future, each mother was consoled by having conceived and the fact of her pregnancy convinced her that she would be able to conceive again. The miscarriage shattered the mother's complacency about her fertility, which changed her outlook for future childbearing by making her feel vulnerable.

Bansen and Stevens's qualitative study is largely endorsed by the work of Swanson (1999) which prepared a 'Human Experience of Miscarriage Model'. This theoretical model demonstrates the stages of the woman's experience beginning with 'Coming to know', through 'Losing and gaining', 'Sharing the loss', 'Going Public', 'Getting through' to 'Trying again'.

The grief associated with miscarriage is beginning to be more widely recognised and researched. In their work on follow-up to miscarriage, Nikcevic and colleagues found that, even though one-third of women could be given no reason for their loss, anxiety was significantly reduced in those women attending for follow-up (2000). These researchers consider that the information obtained helped the woman to assume some control over her life. Nikcevic and colleagues' focus on anxiety resonates with the observation by Rowsell and colleagues that anxiety escalates in women with recurrent miscarriage, rather than the reverse (2001). These women's anxiety levels reach such a level as to be comparable with post traumatic stress disorder. The possibility that allocating the woman some control over her experience, in the hope that her grief may be facilitated, is now gaining wider acceptance (Ankum *et al.*, 2001).

Ritual and recognition

With the help of self-help organisations, the problem of creating ritual to mourn a miscarried baby is beginning to be addressed (SANDS, 1995). In spite of these encouraging developments, Lovell still finds it necessary to argue that 'there is a need for the recognition of the dead baby as a person and for the legitimation of mourning' (1997: 41). The need for such legitimation is evidenced by the fact that the registration of a miscarried baby is not a legal requirement nor is burial or any other ritual. Appropriate documentation, though, may be 'greatly valued' by the parents (SANDS, 1995). On the other hand, it has been suggested that parents may resent the need to register the birth of a stillborn baby (Cooper, 1980), even though it constitutes a recognition of their loss.

Termination of pregnancy

UK abortion legislation (1967) makes termination of pregnancy (TOP) not illegal in certain clearly defined circumstances; these include 'social' reasons as well as situations in which there is 'a substantial risk that if the child was born it would suffer from such physical or mental abnormalities as to be seriously handicapped'. When undertaken for the latter reason TOP may be known as termination for fetal abnormality (TFA).

Since this legislation was enacted there has been a plethora of research on the emotional outcomes of 'social' TOP. The lobby seeking to reverse or at least amend the legislation have been not insignificant in initiating such research.

Cultural implications

TOP is contentious and raises many ethical issues. In some countries the legislation is not yet securely in place, which may affect our use of literature from countries such as the USA. We should also bear in mind the effects of certain religious groups whose attitudes to TOP may be carried over into the area of TFA.

Grief of termination of pregnancy

Grief associated with elective termination of an uncomplicated pregnancy (TOP) is problematic. It may be for this reason that it tends not to be included in the research-based literature on grief (Bewley, 1993). On the other hand, guilt following elective TOP is not infrequently addressed (Salladay and Cavender, 1992; Tentoni, 1995; Mpshe *et al.*, 2002). Writing from a US point of view, Carter (2003) clearly demonstrates the way in which data and literature on this topic may be manipulated to support the bias of the author. In view of the frequency with which TOP happens, and the grief which is likely to be engendered, this topic deserves more serious attention. The experience of grief following TOP for fetal abnormality, however, does tend to be recognised and accepted (see page 45).

A detailed account of the experiences of a small number of women having a termination of pregnancy is provided in research by Moulder (1998). She regrets the less individualised care provided for women undergoing a TOP where no fetal abnormality has been demonstrated. This woman's care features 'respectful caution' (1998: 92) rather than genuine engagement. The health care providers tend to assume that the woman is firm in her decision and will make her needs known. This 'hands-off' approach is apparent in the staff's acceptance of the woman's decision, assumption that TOP is only a minor intervention and certainty that the woman is responsible for her well-being.

Another qualitative research project, undertaken in Canada, focused on the woman's experience of unexpected pregnancy (Marck, 1994). This research found that a termination in such circumstances has very different meanings, depending on a range of factors. These meanings were found to bear little relation to the virtually automatic assumptions which the woman encounters in care providers and others.

Just as the research by Marck demonstrated our limited understanding of the meaning of termination to the woman, a counsellor speaks of seeking to help the woman to work out the meaning of her termination. In her account of her counselling role, Everett (1997) emphasises the crucially private nature of a termination of pregnancy. This means that the woman undergoing this operation does not have the support of family and friends, as in other situations of loss. Similarly, Everett reports her unsuccessful attempts to remedy this deficiency by establishing a post-abortion support group. She considers that women's 'acute anxiety about what other people are going to think' prevents them from attending. In her counselling role, Everett aims to help the woman to work out what this decision means for her. She also emphasises the need to accept the woman's feelings and that women are 'entitled to feel relieved' and that feelings of extreme sadness are acceptable too. By way of exemplifying the woman's feelings, Everett reports how one woman had very much wanted to take the fetus home with her, but that she had not felt able to ask whether she could. Thus, for a range of reasons, facilities available to other women who are grieving perinatal loss may be denied to this woman.

Although not focused on grief, a critical literature review illuminates the woman's psychological experiences and sexual relationships after termination of pregnancy (Bradshaw and Slade, 2003). These researchers clearly demonstrate the woman's psychological distress, which decreases after the operation. This decrease, however, may not be as rapid as is sometimes assumed, possibly taking several weeks before the woman regains her equanimity. These researchers identified the relative salience of anxiety, as opposed to depression. Bradshaw and Slade found less research on the woman's intimate relationships, but what was found suggests that TOP, if anything, has an adverse effect.

Termination of pregnancy for fetal abnormality

Whether the general observation, of limited adverse emotional sequelae occurring after 'social' TOP, applies to TFA must be addressed. The situation is crucially different because, when TFA is undertaken, although the pregnancy may not have been planned, the fact that it has continued until the major prenatal diagnosis (PND) procedures are completed after about eighteen weeks suggests that it is wanted.

Decision-making

The series of decisions which may end with the mother grieving the loss of her baby through TFA will have begun some time earlier, possibly before she ever contemplated pregnancy. Whether she is able to take advantage of prenatal diagnosis (PND) depends on high-level policy decisions about whether it is to be available in her locality and whether she meets the criteria laid down, such as a lower age limit for amniocentesis.

The reasons for women deciding to accept PND were explored in an important study by Farrant (1985), which illuminated the conflicting views held by mothers and their medical advisers. She found that mothers seek the 'all-clear' to allow their pregnancies to continue confidently, while the priority for obstetricians is the diagnosis and abortion of affected pregnancies.

The decisions open to mothers may be limited by obstetricians' concern about 'wasting' resources. Some may require a commitment that, should a positive diagnosis be made, the mother will go through with TFA (Richards, 1989: 177). While decisions are assumed to be made on the basis of complete information, this may not always be forthcoming. Farrant's examples include the priority obstetricians give to positive results and the general failure to inform of negative results, expecting mothers to conclude that 'no news is good news'.

Hypothetical decisions were sought by Green and colleagues (1993) in their study of attitudes to PND and TFA in 1,824 pregnant women. These researchers showed that women's unwillingness to contemplate TFA did not prevent them from accepting PND. This apparent contradiction may be explained in three ways. First, these authors suggest that women's lack of understanding of the 'PND package' may prevent them from making the connection between PND and TFA. PND may be viewed as merely hurdles to be overcome to ensure a healthy baby, possibly regardless of test results. There may be an element of magical thinking in this attitude (see pages 36 and 104). Second, Green and colleagues suggest that being informed about the baby's condition may help a woman to prepare for the birth of an affected baby. Third, these researchers endorse Farrant's observation, that first and foremost women seek reassurance, rendering attitudes to TFA of little consequence.

The 'enormous' pressures applied to mothers to go through with TFA have been identified by Rothman (1990); in North America these include, first, financial pressure, by the provision of less state support to people with disabilities. Second, pressure also exists in individual women who may feel guilty at choosing to give birth to individuals who suffer such discrimination. Third, social pressure derives more and more from the view that disability is the direct responsibility of the mother and less as divine or any other intervention.

Breaking bad news

For a small proportion of the mothers accepting PND, it will be necessary for them to be given bad news in clinical situations, such as the ultrasound (US) department. Statham and Dimavicius (1992) discuss how this painful situation may best be handled, reminding us of parents' sensitivity to anything being 'not quite right'. The authors discuss the problem of the technician who is competent to identify a problem but lacks sufficient authority to explain it to the parents. The authors suggest how to handle the seemingly interminable wait to be 'told officially', without aggravating the distress of the parents or those waiting their turn. Jargon is ruled out and viewing the screen to see the problem is recommended to provide maximum information. While the problem of preparing staff to face this challenging task is happening in the paediatric area (Farrell *et al.*, 2001), midwives may be less well prepared (Robb, 1999).

The effect on the developing emotional relationship

PND may affect the development of the mother's love for her baby by resetting her emotional clock in several ways. The mother may not permit herself to love her baby until she has the 'all-clear'. The 'tentative pregnancy'

(Rothman, 1986) puts the emotional relationship on 'hold' pending the results. This relationship may be facilitated by seeing the baby on US scan (Richards, 1989) but, unfortunately, the magical significance of this experience may be wasted on the US technician.

Once the mother has successfully negotiated the hurdles of PND, her 'tentative' stance is shed as she swings into pregnancy mode, allowing herself to bloom. The celebration of a so-called 'negative' result may anticipate, or even supplant, the celebration of the birth.

I have already referred to mothers' limited understanding of PND, having used the term 'all-clear' to describe mothers' interpretation of PND results; this is because of the not uncommon assumption that, because PND has revealed no problems, the baby must be perfect (Reid, 1990: 304). I fear that the mother, having convinced herself of normality, may react particularly badly to a more minor problem, such as an extra digit.

Psychological sequelae

Although some may assume that the woman's only reaction after TFA is one of relief at having avoided the birth of a baby with a handicap, the reality is less straightforward. As with other situations, we assume that, because we don't see the problems, they don't exist. Iles (1989) suggests six reasons why TFA is associated with emotions other than relief:

1 These are wanted pregnancies, as mentioned already.
2 Because TFA is undertaken later, the demise of the pregnancy will be obvious to those around, requiring explanations and risking criticism. Additionally, 'labour' is a longer and more distressing event.
3 Handicaps not incompatible with life produce guilt in the mother for not keeping and coping with the child.
4 The risk of recurrence may threaten future childbearing.
5 In older mothers the chances of successful childbearing may be diminishing.
6 The abnormality in the fetus, conceived by the parents, engenders guilt and lowered self-esteem at the failure of a normal process. Guilt is doubled, on the grounds of failed reproduction and deciding on TFA (Raphael-Leff, 1991).

The difficulty of the mother's grieving following TFA is attributed to the baby being unseen, the lack of a grave, and trivialisation of the mother's loss.

Richards (1989) argues that in this context, as in others, our knowledge is outstripping our ability to use it safely. Although research demonstrates the problems which women may encounter following TFA, it remains to be seen whether our care is able to reduce these problems. One of the problems in this woman's care was investigated by Young and Bennett (2002). The absence of midwives' routine home visiting following TFA demonstrates the limited attention given to this woman's physical and emotional well-being. Her care was found by Rillstone and Hutchinson to present further prob- . lems in a subsequent pregnancy (2001). The couple became defensive and resisted emotional attachment to the developing baby. On the other hand, though, they developed dependent relationships with health care providers and couples sharing similarly painful experiences.

The newborn with a handicap

The concerns commonly experienced by the pregnant mother may not prepare her for the reality of her baby being born with an unexpected handicap (Niven, 1992). The maternity staff need to understand the extent of the adjustments which are required of her if she is to love and care for her baby. Some may think that, because of PND, no babies are born with unexpected disabilities. But, perhaps because of the machinery being used, the human being using it, or the mother not availing herself of PND, babies may still be born with unexpected handicaps (Chitty *et al.*, 1991).

Terminology and definition

The terminology used to describe this baby varies hugely. While avoiding any suggestion that a baby with a handicap is deficient, it is essential to emphasise their difference from other babies and from the baby which had been expected. For this reason and recognising its limitations I, like Niven, use the terminology which parents are likely to understand and use.

In thinking about handicap I include a wide range of problems which become apparent neonatally. They may be more or less serious and have a similarly wide variety of implications for the baby and her family. Although the mother's reaction is likely to follow a certain pattern, the depth and duration of her response will vary according to the meaning she attributes to this baby and to the handicap. I look at the situation when the baby's survival is uncertain in Chapter 8.

Grieving

The response to handicap is essentially similar to the grief reaction in other situations. This mother needs to grieve the loss of the perfect baby about whom she had fantasised, and to end that relationship (Solnit and Stark, 1961). Overpowering emotional demands are placed on her by the need, at the same time, to come to accept and grow to love her real baby with the handicap. She may develop feelings of unreality due to uncertainty of who the baby is: whether she is the perfect baby being mourned or the real baby who needs loving care and attention.

Denial may feature prominently in this mother's grief, as in a mother I cared for whose baby showed features of Down's syndrome. We informed her of the likely diagnosis and she assured us that 'He looks just like his Dad'. It was interesting to find that her observation was correct, but investigations confirmed the diagnosis, by which time she was coming to know and love her son.

Another significant feature of this mother's grief is her occasional feeling that her child might be better off dead (Lewis and Bourne, 1989). Such thoughts are alarming. They aggravate the feelings of guilt which grief invariably carries with it and may give rise to a true depression. Perhaps parents should be warned that these guilt-provoking thoughts will emerge, in the hope that the mother will not be too frightened by her own feelings.

Because of her perception that grief is inappropriate, the mother may never complete this task. Her relationship with her real baby is, therefore, unable to become established and her grief may reappear unpredictably with future losses (see Chapter 7).

Breaking the news

The circumstances in which the parents learn of their child's handicap will vary according to its nature, but the method of being told is viewed critically. Dissatisfaction with the way the information was given among parents of babies with Down's syndrome is clear (Cunningham *et al.*, 1984). This study also shows that this is not simply a case of 'shooting the messenger'.

Looking to the future

Because a baby is perceived as comprising the characteristics which the mother values most highly in herself (see page 17), the birth of a baby with a handicap represents an additional narcissistic insult to her self-esteem (Leon, 1990). This feeling may be aggravated by the child being an ever-present reminder of both the parents' loss of their perfect baby and their own failure (Raphael-Leff, 1991).

The parents' feelings of guilt and the likelihood of recrimination and blame within the relationship emerged in my recent study. A midwife recalled a mother who had just relinquished her Down's syndrome baby for adoption at the insistence of her husband:

MARIE: . . . maybe she was frightened to come and see the baby in case she did form an attachment to the baby and took it home it would end her marriage. If, you know, at the end of the day if she takes that baby home she might end up losing her husband. She's left with one child, an abnormal handicapped child, to cope with as well, and no husband.

Relinquishment

Although it is widely accepted (Sorosky *et al.*, 1984; Woodger, 2000) that grieving following relinquishment has many features in common with grieving loss through death, there are certain crucial differences. The data from my own qualitative study (Mander, 1995b) suggest that, as in any grief, there is a capacity for deviation from the general pattern. Certain deviations which may impede grieving appeared regularly among the mothers I interviewed, leading to the conclusion that there is scope for intervention to benefit this mother.

Delay in grieving

Delayed grieving may be regarded as a pathological state, possibly associated with a voluntary avoidance of the pain of loss. For a small number of the relinquishing mothers the voluntariness was clear:

IONA: OK, so I grieved when I was in hospital. I cried nearly all week. . . . But I think you can't just shut off something like that . . . completely, which is what I tried to do.

The extent to which the delayed grieving experienced by relinquishing mothers is voluntary must be questioned as many appear to have had some external pressure applied to 'conform' in the interests of secrecy and to benefit the family:

BARBARA: Because I had had to go from the hospital home, the circumstances . . . having to pretend that nothing had happened and in effect not being allowed to mourn. I hadn't been allowed to do any of this.

Relinquishment usually happens while the woman is relatively young, so that her life soon becomes filled with events that may impede her grieving. These events may involve family responsibilities:

HILDA: It's getting worse now because I had the boys to think of, so that kept it in the background. Now the boys are grown up, I think more now. I was busy with them and it's hurting worse now.

Work-related factors may also serve to have a similar delaying effect. Occasionally, work was regarded by the mother, with help from those near her, as therapeutic in dealing with overt grief. Some, like Jessica, soon realised that the therapy she had been recommended was merely papering over the cracks:

JESSICA: I had no outlet and so there are lots of feelings which have never been let out. The main thing was to get back to work.

It is clear that, for the relinquishing mother, her grieving is suspended while she, with the connivance of others, gets on with her life. The reactivation of her grief when her life is less busy is a shock, although there is another factor which exacerbates the grief when it does manifest itself.

Being unable to share grief

In emphasising the 'shared' nature of grief, Clark (1991) raises the inevitability of death for all of us and thus the community experience in which the bereaved person is nurtured and sustained by those around. It may be that relinquishment is perceived as a deviant form of behaviour in a society, such as the UK, where the prevailing pattern is for every mother to care for her own baby. This perception of being deviant and being stigmatised, described by one mother as 'shame', was strongly felt by some mothers:

URSULA: I think that a hospital is there to give care to people, not a court room where you are judged for what you have or have not done. This midwife did this, because when she read my notes her attitude to me changed. She had been kind and welcoming when I came into the labour ward, but after she read them she was chilly. I asked her 'Have you read my notes now?' She said 'Yes'.

This perception was also reported by some midwives:

GAY: I think secrecy's quite important for certain people, yes. If it was a concealed pregnancy and then they want to go back and – because for some people unmarried mothers are still – especially out in the country it seems to be very much frowned upon. Yeah. I don't really think we are as permissive as all that. I think people like to think we are, but I don't think we are.

Jones (1989) discusses grief in the context of another group, gay men, who may be stigmatised or regarded as deviant, though he prefers to discuss the 'absence of recognition' of their relationship. Because the relationship is not sanctioned by society the bereaved partner may not be offered the support usually available to the bereaved person and, Jones maintains, their grief work may be inhibited. If the relationship of the relinquishing mother with her baby is similarly unrecognised, she may find herself not only being isolated from this essential community support but possibly additionally being stigmatised for her deviant behaviour in parting from her baby. This silent isolation was clear:

KARA: I found it really hard to adjust myself back into a normal . . . it was like mourning a bereavement. It is like somebody's died but when somebody dies it is different because it is talked about.

To Clark the significance of the funeral is fundamental: 'While we have been robbed of relatedness and are threatened with brokenness, through coming together to remember and to honour the person who has died, we affirm the vitality of our bonds with others' (1991).

Although a funeral is accepted and expected if a baby dies perinatally, the mother who relinquishes has no equivalent rite of passage:

DEBRA: On the day when I gave her up I dressed her ready for the adoptive parents. My parents and me were sitting in a bare room and I had planned what I would do when I handed her over, adjusting her shawl and everything. Then the social worker came and said 'I'll take your baby now' and she did. I was unable to do any of the things I'd planned – no ceremony, no kiss or anything. It's the hardest thing I've ever done. I'll never get over it. (TEARS)

A decidedly assertive mother who relinquished her baby more recently was able to arrange the ceremony which she wanted:

OLIVIA: My parents are Mormons and . . . I arranged for our church leader to come in and bless her. I felt that this was appropriate. We had to go into the [ward] utility room to do it. My flatmate was there and her boyfriend and my younger brother. It was not really a goodbye ceremony; it was more a way of recognising her as my child that is a part of me to go to Christian parents. The blessing was my way of establishing the baby's rights as an individual, a way of recognising the break from being mine. The blessing was the right thing to do . . .

'Letting go'

Walter (1999) suggests that even in normal, healthy grieving it may never actually be possible to 'let go' of the one who dies. He suggests that the integration of memories may better describe the final stage of the grieving process. If this is so, it raises the question of whether there is any possibility of the relinquishing mother ever completing this stage of grieving in view of her profound awareness of the possibility of the physical reappearance of the relinquished one. The work of Bouchier and colleagues (1991) establishes the widespread prevalence of the desire to resume contact with the one who was relinquished and touches on the effect of this desire on the mother's grieving. The mothers in my own study were all aware of the possibility of future contact:

JESSICA: I often think about the possibility of my child trying to trace me and make contact . . . .

It is clearly apparent that, for the mother who relinquished her baby, the possibility, even hope, of future contact is genuine. Some mothers demonstrated a real awareness that the lack of a conclusion to the relationship impedes complete grieving:

LENA: But sometimes I think when you're young and you have them adopted it's like a death – it's a bereavement when you lose it, y'know. But if you lose somebody through death, you know that that's them gone. When you give up your baby you know that it is somewhere else. Sometimes, I wish she had died; then I would know that I'd see her again.

These comments would appear to reinforce the observation by Bouchier and colleagues (1991): 'The balance between loss and hope is a difficult one for all human beings to maintain.'

Non-completion of grieving

Despite definite similarities between relinquishment and loss through death, which indicate that relinquishment is a form of bereavement, lack of any conclusion impedes the resolution of grief due to relinquishment.

Infertility

Grieving a child may seem inappropriate in a couple who have not even been able to conceive. Such uncomprehending attitudes aggravate the feelings of the infertile couple. In this section we consider whether grief is relevant in this context and, if so, the factors which may affect the couple's grief.

Definition and incidence

When we discuss 'infertility' we tend to assume the 'involuntary' prefix; I am discussing involuntary childlessness, rather than voluntary infertility which results in the couple being 'child free'. Although occasionally defined as the inability to have the number of children which they desire, infertility is ordinarily defined in terms of the duration of unprotected sexual inter-course without conception, usually one year, but when the couple seeks help will vary according to factors such as their age, life style and cultural background.

The incidence of infertility varies according to the criteria which are used to define it, but the usual estimate is that about 15 per cent of couples are childless. The majority of couples who consider themselves infertile have not had any children, but over 33 per cent of couples who are investigated for infertility are having difficulty conceiving a second or subsequent child (Dor, 1977).

Responses

Frank (1984) describes the grief of the infertile couple as relating to an abstract or potential loss rather than the tangible loss which has featured to a greater or lesser extent in the other forms of loss which I have considered. Theirs is not the actual but the potential loss of their child, their childbearing experience and being parents. They grieve not only their lack of a child, but also their loss of genetic continuity and their loss of fertility (Menning, 1982). The fact that this is a totally abstract loss does not facilitate the couple's grieving and may make it more difficult (Frank, 1984).

Although this couple's grief has much in common with the grief which we know happens in many settings, it also has certain unique features. First, the realisation of an infertility problem dawns on the couple as a total surprise (Menning, 1982). We are accustomed to assuming that we are fertile and to taking the appropriate action to control, or rather limit, it. This assumption continues into the area of childbearing, which we may blithely assume will happen when contraception ceases. Ironically, at this point the realisation dawns that the contraceptive precautions were unnecessary. Callan and Hennessy (1989) draw our attention to the perception of a lack of or loss of control over their lives which compounds the grief of infertile people. These relatively unfocused aspects of the grief arising from infertility are explored in terms of their public and private nature in a qualitative research project (Kirkman, 2001).

The second factor which is unique to the grief of an infertile couple is the 'psychological roller-coaster' (Frank, 1984). Usually a person who is grieving experiences distress which gradually, despite some oscillation and either healthily or otherwise, is resolved and allows the person to continue her life. Because infertility and its investigations and treatment relate closely to the woman's cycle, the grief is regularly exacerbated when her menstrual period reminds her yet again that she has not conceived.

Aggravating factors

There are many factors which may 'rub salt into the wound' of the couple's infertility. The everyday assumptions which I have mentioned already are examples. Similarly, there are the well-meant but potentially cruel reminders from would-be grannies and aunties, which reflect this society's pronatalist attitudes and are referred to by Menning as 'needling'.

Infertility investigations may or may not provide a diagnostic label or indicate the cause of the problem, which in turn suggests a solution. The absence of a diagnosis is the least satisfactory outcome (Frank, 1984). Having suggested that a solution may exist, we should look more closely at the possibility. All too often solutions are no such thing, as many methods of 'assisted reproduction' carry implications which make them unacceptable to one or both of the couple, such as the involvement of a third party in AID, or the lack of babies of a suitable age or ethnic background for adoption, or the under-publicised failure rates of reproductive technologies.

Effect on relationship

In the same way as men and women grieve any form of loss differently, the response of each partner to their infertility is likely to differ and generate tensions within the relationship. The differences which have been identified in grieving perinatal death (see Chapter 7) apply equally in the couple's acceptance of their infertility. It is possible that the resulting conflicts are also similar.

Because in the majority of couples the cause of infertility is attributable to just one of the partners, the other partner may inhibit their own grieving in order to be strong for their infertile mate, raising the likelihood of accusations of being callous or unfeeling and the potential for a deteriorating spiral in the relationship.

The mother with HIV/AIDS

Loss, death and bereavement are very real to a woman with HIV/AIDS. This is partly because of the possibility of her own death having been brought unexpectedly closer, but also because of the likely deaths of friends, lovers and, perhaps, children. To these deaths may need to be added the loss of health, relationships, sex, future, employment, self-esteem, security and independence (Sherr, 1995a; Nord, 1997). Currently, we believe that a fore-shortened life-span faces most people with HIV infection, although the use of antiretroviral medication has served to slow the progression of HIV infection to AIDS and from AIDS to death (Belcher and St Lawrence, 2000).

It is essential to handle data on HIV/AIDS with care, because it is an area in which research and, hence, knowledge is far from complete. Our knowledge about HIV/AIDS is growing daily, though, and much of what we believed to be factually correct in the early 1980s, when these conditions were relatively new, has since been overturned. Examples include the effects of pregnancy on the progression of HIV to AIDS and the rate of vertical or mother-to-child transmission. There are many reasons why statistical information may be less than accurate, including logistic, social and even political reasons. An example is the way that statistics have tended to underestimate the number of women affected, which has been due largely to women's more limited access to health services (Bott, 2000). Unsurprisingly, much of the English-language literature on HIV/AIDS originates in the USA. Predictably this material carries with it a strong North American orientation, which may not be entirely relevant to other societies (Lesser *et al.*, 2003).

Despite impressions to the contrary, conception, pregnancy and childbearing are still major side-effects of heterosexual intercourse. It is unsurprising that an infection spread via intercourse should cause concern for both the baby and the mother, although the former tends to predominate. The woman with HIV/AIDS who chooses to embark on childbearing faces an increased likelihood of experiencing a number of losses. These are superimposed on the already socio-economically disadvantaged position of many of the women affected by HIV/AIDS (Cohan, 2003; McCalman, 2003).

One loss that women with HIV/AIDS seem to face less frequently is the loss of choice about whether to become pregnant. In spite of this, Cohan (2003) seems surprised that the affected woman should have the same family aspirations as her unaffected sister. Further, it is not impossible that the desire for a child may be felt more acutely in a woman who perceives her own life-span to be unnaturally foreshortened by HIV/AIDS. This decision-making process is addressed, albeit briefly, by Sherr (1995a). The woman's childbearing decision may be influenced by her suspicion that, because of her HIV status, the health of her baby may be jeopardised before it is even born. Clearly, the most up-to-date information should be made available to this woman when making childbearing decisions. These data indicate that vertical transmission rates are declining, probably due to more effective forms of treatment. The circumstances in which perinatal transmission becomes more likely should be clarified and these are recognised as including factors such as prolonged rupture of membranes and pre-term birth (Cohan, 2003).

While the risk of vertical transmission may be receding, there persists the real risk of a relatively poor perinatal outcome (Brocklehurst and French, 1998). This is clearly a form of loss which the woman should take into account when contemplating pregnancy. These researchers found that the increased risk of infant death is particularly significant in developing countries, but that the increased risk of miscarriage may apply more generally.

A loss which may threaten childbearing women generally is the loss of choice about whether to undergo HIV testing. In the UK a system of 'opt-in' operates, through which the woman is routinely offered testing and she chooses whether to accept it in view of her circumstances (Campbell and Bernhardt, 2003). The argument is being strongly advanced elsewhere that this choice should not be available (Cohan, 2003). Cohan argues that universal HIV testing is necessary and that an 'opt-out' system should be implemented. This would mean that the woman would need to decline this particular test in the 'battery' of prenatal investigations (2003: 201). This proposal would involve the loss of choice for all childbearing women in the interests of those who are affected by HIV. In spite of this proposal to change the approach, even Cohan would admit that compulsory testing is not yet possible. It is possible that the fundamental ethical principles of autonomy and its manifestation in health care as informed consent may be under threat in this debate (Walter *et al.*, 2001).

A further loss which this woman is likely to encounter is her lack or loss of control over her hoped-for healthy and physiological childbearing experience. Because of the known and suspected risks for the woman and her baby she will be the focus of considerable medical attention throughout her childbearing and childrearing years, which is unlikely to have been anticipated or sought after. This loss of the satisfaction of completing childbirth physiologically applies not least to the birth. The finding that transmission is markedly reduced by the administration of zidovudine and nevirapine and the birth of the baby by elective caesarean are likely to serve to determine the woman's experience (Brocklehurst, 2004).

For the HIV/AIDS-affected woman in a developed setting, a further loss may be found in the recommendation that she should not breastfeed her baby. This is yet another situation in which it has been assumed that transmission of HIV from the mother to her baby occurs (Cohan, 2003; CHI, 2004). For this reason, the woman's anticipated enjoyment of the experience of providing sustenance for her child would be denied her. This experience, to which Western society currently attaches so much significance, would have to be foregone (Macrory, 2003). The recommendations for the woman living in a less-developed setting, though, are less clear due to the well-known risks inherent in bottle feeding (CHI, 2004). The 'no breastfeeding' dogma has been seriously questioned by Coutsoudis and her colleagues (2001). This prospective study was undertaken in Durban, which may be regarded as a *relatively* developed society. This study encouraged women to choose their infant feeding method, but women who chose to breastfeed were expected to do so exclusively. The other two groups of women either only bottle-fed or practised mixed feeding. The practice of exclusive breastfeeding is regarded as significant in the finding of no difference in HIV transmission between the three groups.

The mother may be concerned that she may lose the satisfactory outcome of her childbearing experience. This is because she may not be in a position to see her child's healthy growth and development. This may be through her own morbidity or mortality or that of her child. Such a concern is becoming less relevant in developed countries. In less-developed countries, the effect of HIV/AIDS on the woman and/or her baby makes this concern much more real.

Summary

This chapter began by examining the features which serve to make loss in childbearing unique. I then moved on to apply this knowledge to real life by looking at a range of childbearing situations which include a significant element of grieving. I have not been able to consider here what some may regard as the 'minor' or short-term griefs which are associated with a wrong-sex baby, a wrong birth or the loss of the fantasy or ideal baby. I have shown that there are many common features in these grieving situations, but there are also factors which are unique to each and which have implications for the care which is provided.

5 Caring for the grieving mother

In the last chapter we explored the features of perinatal loss which may adversely affect the mother's grieving. Some of these features apply across the range of different forms of loss, whereas others are unique to specific situations. In this chapter we look at the implications of this knowledge for the care of this mother. It is necessary to bear in mind that her care may be happening at any stage in her loss. It may be as early as when she suspects or realises that loss is imminent or it may be as late as during a subsequent pregnancy and birth.

An approach to care

This chapter looks, first, at general issues which influence care, before focusing on to the principles which determine any interventions when providing care for this mother. In this chapter I take a conceptual approach, looking at issues and principles, as I noted in the Introduction, in order to avoid checklists or a cookbook format. It is sometimes suggested that checklists do have a place in the care of the grieving mother; they have been recommended in order to provide 'direction', although whether 'direction' is an obligatory instruction or an advisory suggestion remains unclear. Instruction may be appropriate when relatively junior staff find themselves providing care in situations for which they are inadequately prepared. Alternatively, a checklist may be a useful method for informing other members of staff of what has been achieved with the grieving mother, to avoid her having to repeat the same information at each change of shift.

There is a danger that checklists may start out as helpful direction or guidance, but may become prescriptive 'tablets of stone', the meaning of which is long forgotten (Lewis and Bourne, 1989). Similarly, checklists may result in a production-line approach, serving as a barrier to open caring and protecting staff from painful psychological interaction (Menzies, 1969). Cautioning us to be wary of 'how-to' approaches to this mother's care, Leon (1992) recognises the place of general guidelines, but fears that they may inhibit 'emotionally engaging [with] parents'. As with many aspects of care, a routinised approach, which a checklist generates, denies the uniqueness of both the mother's grief and the care which may be offered to her. I would argue strenuously, that what is becoming known as the 'checklist culture' has no place in the care of the grieving mother.

Avoiding a prescriptive approach is one reason for focusing on the principles influencing this mother's care. Additionally, the principles of care are relatively unchanging, while our provision of care may be affected by any number of factors, such as the individuals involved, the meaning they attach to the loss, and the local circumstances.

The aims of care

When deciding how to offer care to this mother, it is necessary to ask first what we are trying to achieve. It is essential to take a long-term view of her care, so I suggest that the aim should be to help her to initiate mourning and to minimise any impediments to grieving. In this way, care should help her to recover as healthily as possible from her loss.

General principles underpinning care

There are certain general principles which are applicable to many aspects of care but which assume particular significance in this context. We should consider these before moving on to think about those principles which are unique to our care of the grieving mother.

Honesty and directness

The staff who are responsible for giving information about potential or actual loss may be tempted to skirt the issue in the hope of breaking bad news 'gently'. This sadly misguided intention is likely to result in compounding the mother's confusion, rather than clarifying matters. The mother seeking to have her worst fears either confirmed or refuted deserves this information with the minimum of delay. Although some may argue that 'a little delay' may be acceptable, I cannot imagine how this benefits the mother. Whether the mother is made to wait 'to be told' pending the arrival of her partner should not be an issue if she is well supported during and after the giving of the bad news (Statham and Dimavicius, 1992).

Who cares?

Whether the grieving mother should be cared for by staff specialising in bereavement is an extension of the argument discussed in Chapter 6 on counselling. A Bereavement Support Service (Horsfall, 2001) has been developed in some centres but the benefits of such specialised care to the mother are so far unevaluated. While surmising the advantages of care by highly knowledgeable bereavement specialists, it remains uncertain whether these outweigh the security of continuity and ongoing contact with 'kent faces'.

Cultural implications

Because our attitudes to death are inextricably bound up with our culture, it is essential to ensure that the help which is offered is culturally appropriate. In this context culture includes psychological, social and religious perspectives. Caring for a grieving mother is never easy for staff, but the difficulties are aggravated for staff who do not even share her cultural background.

Degree of 'Westernisation'

Although care providers may assume that a certain appearance carries with it particular characteristics, our attention is drawn to the huge variation in 'Westernisation' among a sample of Asian women in south-eastern England (Katbamna, 2000). Assumptions often prove unfounded, but may be maintained in the form of 'generalisations' and 'stereotypes' (2000: 11–12). In the same way as 'Westernisation' varies, adherence to religious and traditional cultural values varies between individuals, requiring us to learn the preferences of those for whom care is being provided. Katbamna clearly demonstrates the differences in value systems between the ethnic groups which form her sample as well as between the individual members of those groups.

Language

In their sample of mothers in east London, Woollett and Dosanjh-Matwala (1990) found that equal proportions (41 per cent) spoke either 'extremely fluent' or 'little or no' English. Perhaps in support of this earlier finding, Katbamna showed that one group of mothers criticised the lack of detail in the informational literature provided in the maternity unit, whereas another group cited 'language problems' as the reason for not accessing information (2000: 68). Although our difficulty with others' languages is often a problem, in a grieving situation when verbal communication is fundamental it becomes crucial. The limited availability of translation aids and interpreters may reflect attitudes endemic in UK society (Phoenix, 1990).

Cultural assumptions

It may be difficult for us to recognise that some of the assumptions which we make about certain aspects of our lives, such as the relationships between men and women, may be little more than that. It may be hard to accept others' views and attitudes, if they differ. This may be a particular problem for those of us who live in areas where we infrequently meet people from ethnic minorities. This became apparent to me when I was caring for a mother whose two-day-old daughter died unexpectedly. The mother explained to me that ordinarily she would have found comfort by reading her Koran, but this was forbidden due to her being 'unclean'. For the same reason she was unable to attend her daughter's funeral, which generated non-comprehension and antipathy among some staff.

Our limited understanding of other ethnic groups emerged in my study of relinquishment (Mander, 1995b), when midwives gave me their impressions of some mothers' attitudes to loss:

MARIE: They have completely different attitudes and things. Nobody understood [a bereaved mother's] need to grieve for this baby because with their religion it is completely different. They completely forget it and say 'Allah has taken it away and I'll be here to have another one.'

Ritual

Distinguishing religious observance from cultural ritual is neither easy nor necessary. Each of the major religions has significant rituals relating to caring for the deceased and for the grieving family. These rituals carry meaning and provide much-needed help and support (Roberts, 2003). It may be necessary to consider the washing and clothing of the body, the timing/form of the funeral, the prescribed mourning/social support, the acceptability of staff of other/no religion and the tolerability of a post-mortem.

Communication

The importance of communication with the mother and in facilitating some of the processes of grieving is examined later, but the significance of this aspect of the care of the grieving mother can not be overstated. The carer's ability to listen may be more important than the ability to talk, but the mother does need to be given information about a range of topics about grieving as well as more mundane matters. How this information is given will determine whether it is accepted and implemented, so the information-giver must be constantly looking out for verbal and non-verbal cues which indicate acceptance or otherwise. It may be helpful at the beginning of a discussion to review topics covered previously. Assumptions relating to the meaning of the pregnancy and its loss are best avoided. While we may correctly assume that her loss constitutes an incapacitating tragedy, there may have been an element of ambivalence at some point in the pregnancy which, after the loss, engenders guilt and which may be magnified disproportionately by our well-meant comments.

Communication with other staff for their benefit is discussed in Chapter 10, but I focus here on communication between staff for the mother's benefit. As I have mentioned already, staff taking over the mother's care at a shift change need information about topics which have been discussed with her.

Better continuity may be achieved through using the concept of primary nursing or team midwifery, to reduce the number of new relationships which the mother is obliged to build. But, regardless of how it is achieved, continuity and consistency of care are crucial.

Communication between staff is additionally important to protect the mother from the painful situations which may arise when staff are ignorant of her loss. I can vouch that the pain is mutual, as I found when I answered a bell in a hectic labour ward to find a newly arrived mother in the throes of giving birth. I helped appropriately, but was perplexed when she burst into tears on finding that she had given birth to a boy. The father patiently explained that they had shared the birth of a stillborn boy two years earlier. Her painful memories were being resurrected, while I felt anger and guilt at being so inadequately prepared.

Lapses of interstaff communication are apocryphal and the consequences dire. Examples would include a bereaved mother being asked where her baby is. In my study, the relinquishing mothers frequently informed me of such lapses and their resulting sorrow. My label 'cock-ups' is entirely appropriate. Aline, a poorly supported thirty-year-old, experienced a cock-up shortly after learning that she was pregnant:

ALINE: The student midwife read my notes which said I was devastated. She asked me how I was feeling and held my hand. She couldn't find the fetal heart using the monitor, so she got the sister. The sister bounced in saying 'What a lovely surprise' and 'Wasn't I pleased?' The student silently pointed to something in the notes and the sister looked aghast. She found the heartbeat and left – fast.

Midwives' need for feedback from mothers on what goes right, as well as wrong, emerged in my study of relinquishment:

OTTILY: You don't get any feedback about how they get on afterwards.
POLLY: We did get a postcard from a bereaved mother who was extremely withdrawn and upset when she lost her baby. But she came to terms with it in a matter of a few months.
ANNIE: The study day . . . was really excellent. Mums came back to talk about it and this provided us with feedback which we don't often get. We usually just get their appreciation at the time and then maybe a letter of thanks a wee while later.

It is clearly necessary for us to learn more about how mothers perceive the care which is provided. It may be that the return visit to discuss the loss may be an opportunity for staff to glean comments about the woman's perceptions of her care.

Principles underpinning care to facilitate grieving

There are certain tasks which, it has been suggested in the research and other literature, facilitate the mother's grieving. The role of carers is to assist her in making progress with these tasks.

Recognising that she has had a baby

Although the research by Davidson is rather old (1977, see Chapter 4) it still provides a useful framework for addressing the mother's confusion about who or what she has lost, as this confusion may impede her grieving.

Establishing the reality of her baby

The lack of reality of a baby who is 'unknown' in the usual sense is thought to be best resolved by the parents having contact with the baby. Alice Lovell (1997), during a research project involving twenty-two mothers who had lost a baby through perinatal death, found that, of the twelve who saw their babies, none regretted having done so. These mothers were powerfully aware of their emotion-laden experience, but they thought that it was rewarding and appropriate. The ten mothers who chose not to see their babies described their feelings as being 'in limbo' and their recollections featured regret.

Hermione Lovell and her colleagues (1986) undertook a small retrospective study of bereaved mothers' views about their care around the time of a perinatal death. Twenty mothers were interviewed for up to ninety minutes approximately three years after their loss. The mothers were still finding difficulty understanding their loss, although those for whom it was their second perinatal loss fared better; their previous experience had taught them the difficulty of grieving for an unknown baby and they resolved to ensure that, at least, their grieving progressed as they wished. These previously bereaved mothers were able to be assertive in making contact with the baby and in arranging the funeral.

It may be argued that women should be able to have an optimal experience of loss without having to lose a second baby in order to do so. But to achieve this, the mother needs to be given information which will allow her to make an informed decision about, for example, making contact with her baby. The information and encouragement about contact which midwives in my study were prepared to give to mothers was variable:

BESSIE: I'd never force anyone though. I certainly would not want to cuddle anything that was dead myself. If that is how she feels she can look at it in the cot and that is fine, or she can look at it the next day and that is fine.

GAY: I think they should see the wee one . . . but they might not think they want to hold it. I think the midwife should really try and encourage them 'cos they'll regret it later on. Y'know, they'll feel it's not really happened to them. But I don't mean that you actually force them to look at it. You know you should just sort of advise them and then it's up to them.

HATTIE: I don't think it's our duty to keep on bringing it up . . . I don't think we should be bullying them into doing what we think's best.

Although the midwives were generally happy to offer some encouragement for the mother to make contact with her baby, they were reluctant to 'strongly encourage' contact.

In his commentary on two case-studies of mothers who had declined contact, Leon (1992), rather than endorsing the orthodoxy of contact, advocates the empowerment of the mother to do what is right for her. He maintains that the helplessness engendered by being forced into certain behaviours may be as painful as any feelings of loss. Leon's misgivings about enforced contact are echoed by Lewis and Bourne (1989) on the grounds that procedures may become unthinkingly institutionalised and devoid of meaning. Like Mallinson (1989) and Bessie (above), these writers plead for the mother to have time to consider and opportunities to reconsider her decision.

This general picture of what may be termed 'sensitive care' of the grieving mother is widely implemented and usually includes some 'encouragement' for the mother to have some contact with her dead baby. In contrast to this general picture, Hughes and colleagues (2002) have undertaken a research project questioning the basis of this encouragement. This prospective study involved sixty-five women who had previously given birth to a stillborn baby (index mothers) and sixty matched controls experiencing their first pregnancy. Quantitative data were collected, from the index mothers; these included, as well as demographic data, details of 'sensitive care' at the time of the stillbirth. Data about the emotional state were collected from both groups of mothers during the third trimester and at one year. These data comprised the Edinburgh Postnatal Depression Scale (EPDS), the Spielberger State Anxiety scale (SSA), the twenty-one-item Beck Depression Inventory (BDI) and the PTSD-1 interview to assess post traumatic stress disorder (PTSD). The Strange Situation Procedure was included in the one-year data collection to measure infant security. These batteries of tests showed that the woman who had chosen to have no contact with her dead baby had significantly lower depression scores than the other women. The woman who chose to see, but not to hold, her baby was less depressed than women who had more contact.

Hughes and colleagues claim that their findings cast doubt on the recommendation that women should be 'encouraged' to have contact with their dead baby. While accepting that 'encouraging' the bereaved mother may not be entirely appropriate, the claims for Hughes and colleagues' study deserve scrutiny. It is necessary to bear in mind that the index mothers effectively chose to which group they would belong; this was not a random sample.

Whether it would be possible to randomise participants in such a sensitive study is difficult to assess. This study does not, however, carry the rigour of a randomised controlled trial (RCT). Further, the relationship between the characteristics measured and unhealthy grieving may not be entirely clear. The researchers assume that high depression, anxiety and PTSD scores indicate unsatisfactory grief, but it is not certain whether these women's grief is dysfunctional, delayed or simply more profound.

The place of the cot

In the course of my research I came to appreciate midwives' need to help the grieving mother accept the reality of her baby and her loss. Although the midwives were keen to encourage contact with the baby and were happy to be open in their communication with the grieving mother, the presence of the cot was regarded with concern, if not distaste. Unlike other equipment which has multiple uses, the cot has only one purpose and that is for holding a baby. This issue was first raised by Irene in response to a question about the birthing room:

IRENE: The cot is always removed from the room before this woman goes in. It would dominate the room if it was present. Even with a couple with a normal healthy baby there is always a comment about the cot when they first go into the room. I would not like keeping the cot in the delivery room. It would probably be too distressing to the parents, although I am speculating about that. There was one woman, though, who refused to hold her baby, so I had to put the baby down on to the trolley while I delivered the third stage. It was really odd having to put the baby on the trolley, I didn't like having to do it. I had to wheel the baby out with all the rubbish. It was so clinical and cold having to put the baby on to the trolley that time.

Clearly the presence of the cot is viewed sufficiently negatively by some midwives to cause them to tolerate much inconvenience to avoid it. As well as its practical use, the presence of the cot assumes a symbolic significance, which may encourage denial in the mother.

KERRIE: I think it's best just to take the cot out. I think it's the right thing to do, possibly because I feel embarrassed in that situation myself. I wouldn't like a cot to be there.

Kerrie's discomfort leads us to ask whether the cot usually being occupied by a living baby serves to remind us of our failure in helping this woman achieve successful childbirth? Alternatively does the removal of the cot constitute a denial of the baby's existence and reduce the birth to a mere surgical procedure?

Recognising that her baby has been born

I vividly recall the care of the grieving mother in labour in the 1960s involving the administration of large doses of 'sedative', actually narcotic analgesic, drugs (Curtis, 2000). This regime, feasible because there was no danger of neonatal respiratory depression, was intended to block the mother's memories of the event, probably for the staff's benefit (Hughes *et al.*, 2002; Kohner, 2000).

Remembering this, I become concerned when 'generous' pain relief is recommended (Adams and Prince, 1990). Although I have argued the right of each mother to effective pain control and to feel the amount of pain which she wants to feel (Mander, 1992a), all involved should be clear about the rationale and use the appropriate medication.

If recollections of her experience are blocked for the heavily sedated mother, the mother who gives birth under general anaesthesia has even fewer memories and greater confusion (Lewis, 1976: 619). I would question whether the mother is similarly denied memories and opportunities to help her work through her grief by the prescription of tranquillisers postnatally.

Realising that she is a mother

The limited physical and visual contact between the mother and baby may cause her and others to either forget or deny that she is a mother. Lovell (1997) suggests that the birth and death, being perceived as positive and negative events respectively, may be seen as cancelling each other out and generating a 'non-event'. The result is that she is 'stripped' of her motherhood, which aggravates her feelings of the non-reality of the event. We are able, through our care, to remind her that, although she may not have a baby with her, she has still achieved the status of mother. Thus, 'routine' postnatal care (see page 76) will in this mother assume extra significance, such as the visits by community staff reaffirming her motherhood.

A crucial component of motherhood lies in caring for the baby. By giving the mother opportunities to behave as ordinary mothers do, such as by cuddling her baby and by bathing and dressing her, it will be reinforced that she was able to show her love by mothering her baby, albeit only briefly (Awoonor-Renner, 2000). A physiological process such as lactation (see page 77) may also serve to reinforce her motherhood if she does not have her baby with her, or she may be able to provide breast milk if her baby is dangerously ill in the neonatal unit (Rådestad *et al.*, 1998).

Recognising that her baby has died

The interventions discussed above to confirm that the baby has been born apply equally to helping the mother to recognise that her baby has died. Her recognition will be facilitated by providing full and factual information about her baby's death. Because she may be unable to take in all the information when it is first provided verbally, it should also be given in writing to allow her to return to it and review what she was told. The reality of the death will be recognised by the use of the rituals which ordinarily happen when death occurs in her culture, such as caring for the body, mourning, funeral rites and providing or ensuring social support.

Creating memories

The significance of memories is clear in the writing of Allingham (1952): 'Mourning is not forgetting, it is an undoing. Every minute tie has to be untied and something permanent and valuable recovered and assimilated from the knot.' Much of our grieving depends on having memories on which we can focus our thoughts, either alone or together, in order to adjust our view of the person who is lost. We come to terms with our good, and perhaps less good, recollections of them, while accepting that we have no more opportunities to interact with them directly. In this way we can grieve and eventually achieve some degree of resolution to our loss. In the absence of tangible memories, any focus for our grief is lacking, which may inhibit its progress.

Ritual

The interventions which we use to help the mother create memories on which to focus her grief are mentioned by Rådestad and colleagues (1996a). They comprise largely the rituals ordinarily associated with death, such as laying out the body, viewing the body and holding a funeral; the burial or cremation serves both to help create memories and to give a physical focus to help long-term grieving. Lewis and Page (1978) describe the interventions they used to create memories of her stillborn son for a mother with pathological grief due to failure to mourn. They reconstructed the 'non-event' by 'bringing the baby back to death' to enable the mother to remember and belatedly grieve her loss. Carers in the maternity area aim to promote healthy grieving by creating memories as the birth and subsequent events unfold. This is preferable to having to intervene retrospectively to resolve pathological grief.

Tangible, durable mementoes serve as a focus for grief as well as confirming the reality of the event. One example, pictures, have long been helpful to bereaved families (Mander and Marshall, 2003). That the use of photography in this context is not a modern phenomenon is further evidenced by Figures 5.1 and 5.2, which were produced in 1925. The possibility of the contemporary mother finding a photograph helpful is apparent in Figure 5.3.

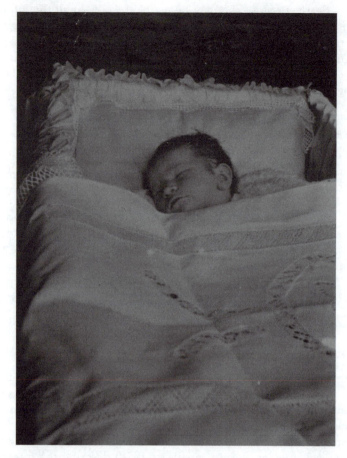

Figure 5.1 Photograph of a stillborn baby (1925)

The baby as an individual

Recognising her as a unique individual helps the mother to differentiate her dead baby from any others and from her own fantasies and narcissistic dreams.

We help her to establish the individuality of her baby by focusing on her unique characteristics as well as the ways in which she differs from any siblings. Even though it is not a legal requirement, the mother may name her lost child, as this provides a focus, as well as helping communication with others. In a situation in which the mother may feel that she has little to contribute, being able to give her baby a name becomes significant, as I learned from the relinquishing mothers in my recent study:

IONA: But Andrea had always been my favourite name and I wanted to give her something and that was all I could give her. So I gave her the name Andrea.

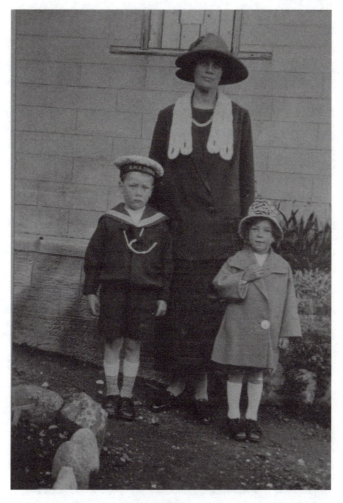

Figure 5.2 The family of the baby in Figure 5.1 during the pregnancy

In a study of perinatal loss associated with the founding of SANDS, Lewis (1978) found that over 60 per cent of her sample of eighty parents considered that having their baby recognised as a real person was their major concern. Giving the baby a name and using her name may facilitate this recognition.

Making the birth as good an experience as possible

Although the possibility of making a perinatal loss into a happy event is remote, it can become at least an experience which the mother is able to recall with satisfaction through having completed it with dignity. To do this the

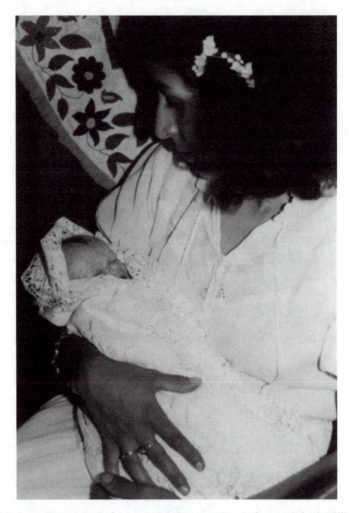

Figure 5.3 A contemporary photograph of a grieving mother with her stillborn baby
(by kind permission of E. Stewart)

grieving mother should be encouraged to participate actively in the birth, as is any mother.

Although, in the past, medication has been used to sedate the grieving mother for the convenience of the staff (see page 66), Dyer (1992) recommends that the mother should, if she wants to, be able to feel the pain of labour. This may correspond with her 'emotional pain' and perhaps also give her as complete an experience of labour as possible. Sensation of her pain may allow her some sense of satisfaction or achievement so that she is able to look back and think 'At least I managed that'.

Fathoming the complexity of this event

The psychological work which the grieving mother faces is overwhelming; she must disentangle and grieve for a confusing mix of potential and actual phenomena. She has to separate out the threads of dreams and reality, of herself and her baby, of this loss and previous and future losses. Completing this mammoth task is helped by sharing the load, and being listened to has been identified as a fundamental need at this time. Kohner (2000) reminds the reader, though, that this is also a very individual need. The mother's difficulty in finding suitable people with whom she may unburden herself needs to be recognised. Senior staff lack the time to spend listening, while younger staff may be considered too inexperienced and not have the personal touch. Family and friends may not be available or may have their own needs (Rajan, 1994).

Effective listening is an important way of reducing the mother's isolation. However, the difficulty of listening to her speaking angrily or guiltily should not be underestimated, especially if her anger is partly directed at carers as it may be hard not to react to what may be perceived as a personal attack.

The difficulty of making time to listen emerged in my study of loss through relinquishment. The midwives told me of the strategies they used to ensure that they were not disturbed while with a grieving mother. They were aware that, although they might make time to be with the mother for an hour, say between 14.00 and 15.00, that might not be the time when the mother felt like 'opening up'. While listening to her we encourage the mother to articulate her dreams about her baby and help her to think about the meaning of her baby and her loss.

She needs to be able to talk about what it is that she feels she has lost without the listener trying to change the subject or backing off. The study by Hermione Lovell and colleagues (1986) found that previously bereaved mothers (see page 24) were able to satisfy their need to talk through their loss. Alice Lovell (1983) draws our attention to a discrepancy which confronts a grieving mother. Ordinarily each of us has some need to communicate with our fellow beings, if only about the weather. But at times of crisis, our need to share our feelings is increased. The grieving mother, however, is faced with the prospect of not even being allowed to satisfy her usual need to talk, let alone her increased 'quota'. This constitutes an 'ironic' discrepancy which may aggravate her feelings of isolation and rejection.

Although we are unable to know what her loss means to her, we assume that it is significant. This enables us to give her opportunities to work out what the meaning is to her. I had to force myself to remember this when I was caring in the postnatal ward for a young mother whose son had been born light-for-dates at twenty-six weeks. She seemed calm, but told me repeatedly that no-one was looking after her dog. She was not keen to see her son. I explained how ill he was and that it was all right for her to be sad. A little while later the neonatal staff asked for her to go to see him and she was able to hold him while he died.

As well as listening, we need to give her information, including telling her that we are available to be there and listen.

Preparing to face the future

Although the grieving mother may have difficulty envisaging a future in the absence of what was a major part of her, we may encourage her to relate her experience of loss to her future life.

Telling her about grieving

By telling her about grieving we are able to help her to understand the process by which she will eventually be able to integrate her loss into her life. Information will help her to know that grief is appropriate, that it is painful, enduring and unique and that her grief may include negative feelings which may shock her. It may be helpful to suggest that such frightening responses have been felt by other grieving mothers. In this way her sense of isolation may be reduced. She should be told, as far as possible, what will and what will not help her grief and be forewarned that the hurtful 'have another' comments are not meant unkindly and are best forgotten. It may help her to know that her experience of loss may change her and those close to her in ways which are unpredictable and possibly unwelcome, but such changes are not unique to grief.

Pitfalls

As well as preparing her to cope with the healthy development of her grief, warnings about certain times and events may prevent her from feeling that she is 'taking two steps back' when they confront her. The widely recognised 'anniversary' reactions may be less than welcome (see below).

The request for a **post-mortem** (autopsy, necropsy) may shock a mother who considers that her baby has been through enough already (Rankin *et al.* 2002). Although this investigation may now, because of certain scandals, be handled more sensitively, the information available to parents still shows room for improvement (DoH, 2003). The possibility of a sensitive approach to this issue is addressed by Forrest (1999), who contemplates the data which may be obtained from a post-mortem and the information which may be given to the parents to show its necessity. She shows that pressurising the parents unnecessarily may alienate them at their most vulnerable time and impair their grieving irrevocably. Forrest mentions the possibility of having to resort to the Coroner's Court or the Procurator Fiscal, indicating that such measures should be used only in extreme circumstances. After a post-mortem the results should always be made known to the parents.

The **funeral** may be regarded as a macabre irrelevance by a young mother with no experience of bereavement and no strong religious faith. An explanation of the likely short- and long-term benefits may help her to decide whether and how it should be organised.

The baby's **nursery** may have been 'dealt with' by well-meaning but unthinking family members but, if not, she may appreciate the opportunity, when she feels ready, to complete this 'unfinished business'.

At **anniversaries** she may be disappointed at her reaction. But when she recollects the joy of, for example, her first scan, her reaction may seem less disproportionate. Others' difficulties are aggravated by some of the anniversaries, such as the conception, being 'hidden'.

Future childbearing (see Chapter 13) should be mentioned to the mother in case she is persuaded, by all the 'have another' advisers, of the need for a 'replacement child'.

Finding support

The benefits of support to those who are grieving have been established in the context of perinatal death (Chambers and Chan, 2004; Rajan and Oakley, 1993; Forrest, 1989) as has the difficulty of resolving grieving in the absence of social support. I look at some issues relating to lay support in Chapter 12.

Being available – The supportive nature of the carer's company emerges in the work of many researchers (Lovell, 1997; Säflund *et al.*, 2004) and I have already observed (see page 60) the need for us to be available for the mother. Our presence may involve listening, information-giving, sharing her tears or just being present. Finding the right balance between being companionable and being intrusive worried the midwives in my study:

KAY: I think that it's a very important thing to give them some privacy. If you're outside with the door open or within shouting distance, they don't need you to be there all the time. A careful decision to make. Also you don't want them to feel that they've just been abandoned – gone away – nobody cares. You've got to tell them 'I'm over the other side.'

The role of the midwife in providing social support for a grieving mother was established in a study of 509 mothers, half of whom had experienced previous pregnancy loss (Rajan and Oakley, 1993). The research midwives gave non-directive social support tailored to the individual mother. This low-tech intervention helped the mothers' emotional health on both a short-term and a long-term basis. The mothers were able to deal with unresolved grief and to prepare themselves to cope with an anxiety-provoking pregnancy. Many of the mothers became more self-confident and reasserted control over their lives.

Family support – Because the family is likely to be providing support on a longer-term basis, they need to be involved in the mother's short-term care and her teaching (see Chapter 7). They also need to understand their own grief as well as hers, partly to help them to avoid well-meant but hurtful comments. In her 1994 study, Rajan found that the other family members may encounter difficulty in providing the support which the grieving mother seeks. Their own needs may predominate over those of the mother, possibly resulting in the nonsensical situation of the mother providing support for those around her. Open and honest communication between family members enables them to share their reactions to their loss; this may happen despite a previously 'closed' system of communication.

Other social support – Family and community support may be forthcoming in the religious or cultural rituals associated with death, such as the funeral.

Like Rajan's (1994) sample, the grieving mothers interviewed by Lovell (1983) found that the 'community' is less caring and comforting than its name implies. This led to the conclusion that the grieving mother might have been better supported if she had remained in the maternity unit longer. The mothers would also have welcomed the support of a self-help group, but only half of the sample were aware that any existed. On the basis of these data, Lovell suggests that the health visitor has an important role to play in the long-term care of the grieving mother.

Being in control

The bereaved mother may feel that her control over her life has been diminished by her loss. This may take the form of learned helplessness, which is a person's response to their own inability to control their circumstances, although whether it occurs will depend on her interpretation of her loss. This term is used to describe the debilitated behaviour of a person who is subjected to some form of assault (such as electric shocks applied in a laboratory) over which they have no control.

Learned helplessness comprises three main components, which are deficits in functioning. First, the deficit in motivation comprises the person's inability to initiate any voluntary responses – on the assumption that to do so would be futile. Second, the cognitive deficit involves the person having difficulty learning at a later stage that responses may produce outcomes. Theirs is the difficulty of unlearning something that they have learned by, possibly literally, painful experience. The third feature of learned helplessness is the depressed affect, resulting from the conviction that you can't do anything about it anyway. These features are based on a view which leads to the expectation that what has happened in the past will continue in the future, that is, their absence of control is not going to change (Garber and Seligman, 1980).

Perinatal loss gives rise to feelings of personal helplessness and pathological grief if the mother believes that there is something she could have done which might have prevented the loss of her baby, such as resting more or eating a better diet. The care which enables this mother to retain both a sense of and actual control relates largely to the information which she is given. Accurate information and possibly a post-mortem report should show her that feelings of self-blame are misplaced. Additionally she needs information about the choices which are open to her and information on which she can base her decisions.

Choices and control – The woman may find herself able to assert control over her experience in one or more of a number of ways. For some mothers induction of labour may be recommended to expedite the birth, and she will decide whether and when this happens (see Chapter 4). There may be a choice about the place where she labours and gives birth, although this may be only the location within the maternity unit; depending on her condition, she may have other alternatives.

I have already considered the mother's decision about contact with her baby (see page 60).

The mother's accommodation after a birth in a maternity unit has been the focus of much attention, although the midwives in my recent study were unaware of the mother's choice:

AMY: The decision is made by nursing staff and hospital policy. Here they always come to antenatal. 'Cos antenatal is the only place with single rooms. But when I worked up at [hospital] they went to postnatal because postnatal had single rooms there and they were a postnatal lady.

HILARY: She has a single room so that she'll be protected from the other mothers.

Hughes's study (1986) indicates that other women were not averse to being alongside a bereaved mother, suggesting that midwives' anxiety about other mothers' actively harmful role is unjustified. These findings are reinforced by the comments of relinquishing mothers who found help among other mothers:

LENA: Actually the women [in the big ward] were OK. And they used to mother me. They realised I was just a kid. They were OK to me. I think before I had the baby I wanted to be in a room on my own. I didn't want anyone to see me. But I was glad really that I was 'cos even though it was [a big ward] the women were all nice. We were all just girls together. They done their exercises and had a bit of a giggle and they all were nice to me. They all sorta looked after me.

These data lead to the conclusion that the grieving mother as well as the other mothers would be happy to share accommodation. The staff who make or at least implement these decisions have other concerns, such as the midwives' anxiety that the grieving mother would be disturbed by babies crying. The midwives were unwilling to contemplate the possibility that this avoidance of other mothers and babies might be associated with a denial of the loss.

The midwives were reluctant to burden the mother with mundane decisions about her care. These decisions include the type of ward in which she is cared for, the size of room which she should occupy or, if larger, the mothers with whom she should share it (pregnant women, new mothers or mothers of babies in NNU). Such decisions were invariably attributed to unit policy. Sharing a room with another mother may be considered to be unhelpful for the grieving mother, as the onset of her mourning is delayed and her support system may be impaired. Midwives' reluctance to allow or encourage the grieving mother to make decisions about her accommodation is unfortunate, as the choices open to her and her control over her situation are being limited.

Lovell (1984) identified feelings of isolation and rejection among her sample of grieving mothers, which related to their being cared for in single rooms. The relinquishing mothers I interviewed referred to themselves as like a 'ghost at the banquet'. Lovell found that hospital staff encounter difficulty in caring for this mother appropriately and as a result transfer her home 'with undue haste'. Although the midwives in my recent study maintained that the grieving mother was in control of how long she stayed in hospital, their examples did not bear this out:

HILARY: I think that as long as everything is all right she should be able to go home the next day. She should have as short a stay in hospital as possible.

LUCY: But we usually tend to let them go home as soon as they want to go home. We would allow them to go home as long as they are physically fit. And that seems to work best as long as we can see that they are coping with the grief as well.

Although lip service is being paid to the mother assuming control, the reality needs investigation. Gohlish's exploratory study (1985) involved interviews with fifteen mothers of stillborn babies to identify the 'nursing' behaviours which were most helpful. Her twenty behavioural statements focused on the mother assuming control over her situation. But those statements which the mothers thought 'most helpful' clearly related to control:

1   Recognise when I want to talk about my baby.
2   Allow me to stay as long or as short a time in hospital as I wish.
3   Let me decide if I want a single room or main ward.
4   Ask me if I want a photograph of my baby.
5   Explain to me that I may produce milk.
6   Explain to me that I can see the baby after several days.
7   Give me pain relief as often as needed.

Grieving mothers felt the need to assume or be allowed more control over their care. Unfortunately my study, which was completed seven years later, fails to show that her findings are being utilised.

Obtaining the care that a new mother needs

As suggested already in the context of care in labour, midwifery care aims to prevent those problems which would create harmful memories and would prevent her focusing her grief on her loss. The need for information, which applies to all mothers, becomes more significant for the grieving mother who is trying to make sense of the confusing situation and conflicting emotions which beset her.

Home visits by the midwife – In view of the haste with which the mother is likely to go home, her care by the community midwife assumes greater significance. Home visits were found to be appreciated for both their physical and their psychological value (Lovell, 1983). These observations contrast with those by Hermione Lovell and colleagues (1986), whose respondents disliked home visits for two reasons. First, the personal characteristics of the midwives were unacceptable, in that they were 'very cut off, very professional'. The second factor, which may not be unrelated, is the difficulty which the grieving mother has in understanding why the midwife visits her, when she has no baby, which would definitely be exacerbated by the midwife being unaware of the mother's loss. Uncertainty about the midwife's role had been encountered by a community midwife I interviewed:

GINNIE: Sometimes they can be a bit antagonistic, you know, the first couple of visits and 'Do you have to come to see me? I don't need a midwife.' And – y'know – if you sit down with them and try and explain that you are there to make sure that she is all right and everything is returning to normal and . . .

Lactation – One of the most helpful nursing behaviours (see page 5) in Gohlish's (1985) study was 'Explain to me that I may produce milk.' A mother may assume that, if she has no baby with her, nothing will be produced with which to feed a baby. Our increasing knowledge of the physiology of lactation shows us that the mother's thought processes are crucially important, so that thinking about her baby has an effect similar to the baby suckling. It is, thus, hardly surprising that the grieving mother produces milk, as recounted by one of Lovell's respondents:

FIONA: Walking down the road and seeing a pram with a baby in it, I'd have to go home and change my tee shirt. It'd be soaked. The milk kept coming for months after.

Fiona seemed to regard her lactation negatively, but we must question whether this need invariably be the case. It may be comforting for the mother to know that, had her baby survived, she would at least have been well nourished. Rådestad and colleagues also suggest that non-pharmacological methods of lactation management may facilitate grieving for this woman by helping her to confront the reality of the death of her baby (1998: 116). These researchers go on to draw attention to the number of bereaved mothers who encounter adverse side-effects from the use of pharmacological methods of lactation inhibition. Although these researchers do not suggest it, it is necessary to question whether such complications may also adversely affect the woman's healthy resolution of her grief.

Summary

Much of the literature reminds us of the bad old days when the 'rugger pass' technique of surreptitiously 'whisking' (Lovell, 1997) the baby out of the mother's presence prevailed. In thinking about our care of this mother we must be wary of forcing a new, perhaps more liberal, orthodoxy on her (Lewis and Bourne, 1989). I have argued in this chapter that our role is to facilitate the mother's healthy grieving, which is assisted by her having as positive a childbearing experience as possible to recall. To achieve this the mother should be encouraged to assume some control of her experience, which, in turn, is dependent on her being provided with accurate, evidence-based information about interventions and outcomes. Unfortunately, such information is still incomplete.

6 Bereavement counselling

I occasionally find myself wondering what bereavement counselling is all about. Tschudin provides an answer of sorts by reminding us that its etymological meaning – to give advice – is 'precisely what is *not* intended' (1997: 6). While counselling began with a very precise focus, it may have snowballed to become something of a panacea. In her contemplation of the reasons for the exponential development of bereavement counselling services, Danbury (1996) blames the change in societal attitudes to death during the twentieth century. This change is partly associated with the medicalisation of death through its removal into hospitals. She concludes, though, that the main reason for this growth in the counselling industry is to be found in the secularisation of society: 'the loss of religion results in the loss of mourning rituals, which makes it more difficult for people to cope with death' (1996: 18).

My anxieties about the purpose of bereavement counselling relate to the fervour of the recommendation, the heterogeneity of those who benefit, the wide-ranging activities included and the variety of practitioners, leading to the conclusion that it is 'all things to all people'. In this chapter I consider the nature of bereavement counselling, who is involved and its relevance following perinatal loss. As in the counselling literature, I use the word 'client'.

What bereavement counselling does and does not involve

Bereavement counselling and grief therapy are not easily distinguishable (Cook and Dworkin, 1992), perhaps due to sloppy terminology or, alternatively, to common areas, such as the client having been bereaved. The large area of overlap between bereavement counselling and therapy increases the risk of confusion. The difference is found in the client (Worden, 2003); in bereavement counselling the client is being supported through uncomplicated grieving, whereas grief therapy addresses the problems associated with pathological grief.

Counselling is defined in terms of the source of control in a nursing context, when the counsellor acts merely as a facilitator to help the client identify and 'sort out his or her own problems' (Burnard and Morrison,

1991). Thus, the relative inactivity of the professional is held to be crucial to counselling.

Interpretations, however, may differ from this facilitative role. Bereavement counselling to prevent psychiatric and psychosomatic disorder has been researched (Parkes, 1980; Forrest *et al.*, 1982). Although counselling does not aim to treat pathological grief, it may constitute a primary or preventative rather than a tertiary approach to disordered grieving. Unlike the supportive approaches involved in counselling, tertiary treatment or grief therapy comprises active and significant interventions to bring about emotional and cognitive changes in the client (Cook and Dworkin, 1992).

Evaluation

As with any form of care, if we recommend bereavement counselling we should be certain that the client is given full information about what it is, as well as any side-effects. This information is only available if the intervention has been rigorously researched. In Parkes's (1980) review of authoritative research, he concludes that bereavement counselling services reduce the risk of disordered grieving. Sigmund Freud's contention, that counselling causes more problems than it solves, is not supported by this evidence. The classical experimental design was utilised in the studies to which Parkes refers; people identified as bereaved through official sources were recruited and randomly allocated to either the counselling or the non-counselling group. After counselling was completed, health measures were applied to assess any differences.

Cameron and Parkes (1983) used a similar design to research the effects of bereavement counselling; they found similarly effective results, but were implicitly critical of this design. These researchers regretted their inability to identify which components of the counselling programme were effective. We may criticise the use of the classical experimental design in more general terms, to the extent that these studies do not establish whether the actual counselling made any difference, because the fact of some intervention may have been sufficient to produce the favourable results. At such a vulnerable time the bereaved person may be grateful for any form of human contact, whether or not it helps her adjustment to her loss. Such alteration in the subject's behaviour because of her involvement in a study, or Hawthorne effect (Porter and Carter, 2000: 27), could have been avoided by amending the design. If, instead of having only two groups of subjects, the researchers had introduced a third 'other intervention' group, they would have been able to ascertain whether counselling was responsible for the improved outcomes. The ethical implications of any such 'other intervention' would need attention, but learning a neutral subject, such as a foreign language, would satisfy the research requirements.

Unlike the other evaluative studies, Forrest and colleagues (1982) focused on the provision of sensitive care in situations of perinatal loss. These forms of care, at the time relatively novel, included the possibility of bereavement counselling. The randomised sample, interviewed longitudinally, comprised twenty-five mothers of stillborn babies and twenty-five whose babies had died as newborns. They found that the intervention mothers recovered from their grief more quickly than the contrast group. The difference was significant at the six-month assessment, but not at fourteen months. As with so many 'packages' of care, though, it is not possible to distinguish the components of the sensitive care provided for the grieving parents in order to demonstrate their effectiveness. Thus, Forrest was unable to establish whether or not bereavement counselling is an effective intervention in perinatal loss.

In her allegedly qualitative study of pregnancy loss, Moulder (1998) reports the dismal experiences of the women in her sample with regard to counselling. A sorry account of 'one-off appointments' and referrals for the bereaved women leads to the bleak conclusion that they 'did not appear to offer them much' (1998: 156–7).

The benefits of these research projects focus on the long-term health outcomes of bereaved people. Little attention is given to the client's experience of counselling, unlike a less authoritative study by Barker (1983) in which general satisfaction and occasional gratitude are reported. This suggestion derives from the attrition rate in Forrest's study, which may have been due to a variety of factors. Only 64 per cent (16) of the supported group and 75 per cent (n=19) of the unsupported group agreed to be interviewed at six months. By fourteen months 40 per cent (n=20) of the original sample were unavailable for interview. Unfortunately we are not told to which group they had been randomised. Although bereavement counselling is not intended to be enjoyable, this loss from the study may indicate dissatisfaction and needs further investigation.

Because the research project by Danbury claims to have focused on the 'effectiveness' of bereavement counselling (1996), it should provide an evaluation of this form of care. The extent to which Danbury achieved these ends is uncertain. Her study involved thirty widowed people who were counselled through a hospice and thirty through Cruse. The refusal rate was low at 10 per cent (n=6). Danbury undertook 'in-depth semi-structured' interviews with the sixty respondents using a pre-coded interview schedule which was analysed by computer. The findings of this study relate largely to the stated satisfaction of the clients and organisational issues which were identified.

Danbury found that a large majority of her respondents thought that their experience of counselling was helpful and that the relationship with the counsellor provided them with good support. Much of her data relate to the events around the death of the spouse, which are questionably relevant. The clients' dissatisfaction with the counsellors emerges in their wish to be able to choose their counsellor, their inability to choose when the counselling should happen and the counsellors' volunteer status. Thus, although Danbury obviously attempted to address important problems, as she herself recognises more research is necessary.

The current vogue for the determination of the effectiveness of any intervention may prove helpful in evaluating the contribution of bereavement counselling. A systematic review undertaken by the authoritative NHS Centre for Reviews and Dissemination (NHS CRD, 2001) investigated the evidence relating to the effectiveness of counselling in treating mild to moderate mental health problems. The reviewers were able to identify only short-term benefits. In the longer term (eight to twelve months) there was found to be no difference in outcomes between counselling and standard care by general practitioners. More recently, a systematic review focusing on nursing inputs for spouses bereaved by suicide or cancer (SEHD, 2004) produced largely similar findings. The SEHD review showed counselling to be ineffective in helping the two main groups. There was, however, sparse evidence to suggest that grief workshops may improve relationships and behavioural difficulties in grieving families.

The client

Clearly, because resources are finite, who receives counselling is determined by what it entails. If counselling comprises non-professional support to maintain healthy grieving, it may be available to many. On the other hand, if it is regarded as a preventive intervention, professionals skilled in psychotherapeutic techniques may be needed, with obvious resource implications.

Worden (2003) suggests indications for counselling; either the person may actually have become 'stuck' in their grief or carers using 'at-risk' criteria may seek to prevent problems occurring. The route by which clients find their way into counselling has been identified as a combination of a 'watching brief' being kept by certain professionals, such as GPs and HVs, and the referral of those identified as being at risk.

The counselling process

While it is neither appropriate nor possible to detail the skills and techniques of counselling here, there are certain essential features which help us to understand it.

The three main approaches which counsellors may utilise are:

- **person-centred**, in which the focus is very much on the present
- **psychodynamic**, in which the effects of past events are addressed
- **cognitive-behavioural**, in which the focus is on learning new techniques and behaviours.

(Macleod, 1993)

The counsellor's 'way of being' incorporates three characteristics (Weston *et al.*, 1998) which may differ from our usual responses to painful situations:

- **Acceptance** means the recognition of the uniqueness of the client's hurt, and being non-judgemental about her feelings.
- **Empathy** comprises the ability to enter the world of the client without the barriers of pity or fear. In their conceptual analysis of empathy Kunyk and Olson (2001) found that it could be regarded as a human trait, a professional state, a communication process, a form of caring, and a special relationship.
- **Congruence** is the self-awareness in the counsellor which allows her to be genuine and accepting of herself. Through her behaviour, she conveys acceptance to her client, as mentioned already.

These characteristics are crucial to effective counselling, as they provide an emotional environment in which healing and growth are nurtured. Although these characteristics may occur naturally in some of us, others may have to learn them during a counselling programme. A supervisor helps a counsellor to maintain these characteristics, ensuring that counselling remains effective.

There are **certain tasks**, in addition to creating an appropriate ambience, with which the counsellor provides encouragement, in order to work through grief (Worden, 2003):

- **Actualising the loss** – through talking about the death and its circumstances and by focusing on tangible manifestations, such as the grave.
- **Identifying and expressing** feelings may be resisted because of the pain which they bring us. The counsellor encourages articulation of anger, guilt, sorrow, anxiety and helplessness.
- **Living without the dead person** may be particularly difficult when roles are complementary and there may be gaps in many aspects of functioning. The counsellor may have to assist practically to show the client her own ability.
- **Relocating the emotions** invested in the dead person helps the client to realise that, although her relationship with the dead person was unique, her emotional energy may eventually be redirected into other, new relationships.
- **By providing time** to grieve, the counsellor helps recognise the gradual process by which we reconcile ourselves to loss. Memories persist in returning and causing emotional reactions for a disconcertingly long time.
- **Recognising 'normal' grief** behaviour means that the client can be reassured that her preoccupation, for example, does not indicate a mental health problem.
- **Continuing support** by the counsellor is within the contract negotiated during the first meeting, although contacts tend to become less frequent before the counselling relationship is due to end.
- **Identifying defences and coping** mechanisms enables the client to work out which are helpful, as opposed to those, such as drugs or alcohol,

which may impair grieving (Worden, 2003). Other differently harmful defences include immersion in work and other forms of denial (Howarth and Leaman, 2001). These defences protect us by diverting our attention away from painful events on a short-term basis, but prevent effective grieving if they persist. Such defensive mechanisms may only be breached if there is confidence in the counsellor.

- **Identifying pathology** and making a referral is necessary when unforeseen problems are encountered. A grief therapist and psychotherapeutic interventions may prevent the difficulty from deteriorating.

The counsellor

Having briefly considered what happens during counselling, it is useful to think about the people who offer this form of help. By way of introducing his literature review, Parkes (1980) lists the three groups of counsellors whose functioning has been evaluated:

1 professional services by trained personnel
2 voluntary services using trained volunteers with professional support
3 self-help or mutual support groups (see Chapter 12).

Although voluntary services contribute hugely to counselling services generally (Danbury, 1996), their input into perinatal bereavement counselling services is less. For this reason I focus on nurses and midwives as counsellors. Although Danbury does not envisage any difficulties (1996: 183), the suitability of nurses and midwives to be counsellors has been questioned. Burnard and Morrison (1991) argue that essential attitudes (see page 179), summarised as 'client-centredness', may not easily fit into traditional nursing thought processes. These researchers surveyed the 'client-centredness' of a mixed sample of 142 qualified nurses. Their opportunistic sample was recruited through attendance at counselling skills workshops. The authors draw attention to the potential unrepresentativeness of the sample, but fail to recognise that, because these nurses were enhancing their counselling skills, they were probably more client-centred in their approach than most nurses. Using an instrument with a maximum score of 70, the nurses assessed their own 'client-centredness'.

The nurses' scores ranged from 22 to 67 with an overall mean score of 39, which Burnard and Morrison interpret as a 'lack of a marked tendency towards "client-centredness" '. They contrast this finding of 'prescriptive' attitudes with the frequent exhortations for patient autonomy. They then suggest that 'client-centredness', because of its reflective approach, may be less than appropriate in a busy clinical setting. The authors do not link their findings to nurses' ability to be 'client-centred' in their counselling, although it is tempting to assume that the attitudes reflected in the questionnaire apply more generally than in the clinical situations which the authors discuss.

Counselling following sudden death

The limited research-based material on bereavement counselling (Robak, 1999) is exceeded only by the absence of research on perinatal bereavement counselling (Redman, 2003). For this reason I draw here on research on counselling in the event of sudden death, which has some aspects in common, such as untimeliness. In an account of a bereavement counselling service in an accident and emergency department (A&E), the nurse-counsellor's educative function is emphasised, as is her ongoing support of relatives at risk of complicated grieving (Yates *et al.*, 1993). The nurse-counsellor provides emotional support for her colleagues, a group of other senior nurses who have been trained to offer a similar service. Yates and colleagues suggest that, in contrast to the findings of Burnard and Morrison (1991), nursing support may be appropriate in bereavement.

Woodward and colleagues (1985), using a social work perspective, recount the counselling service which they established for parents losing a child through SIDS. As with Yates and colleagues (above) the service originated in A&E. Woodward and colleagues describe the importance of the initial assessment in helping parents sort out a range of mainly practical problems. Unlike Yates though, Woodward recommends that appointments be made for home visits, because of the tendency of young bereaved families to avoid their home. Longer-term counselling focused largely on family problems such as marital difficulties and helping surviving children. As observed already, the children who were most seriously affected were those whose parents were coping less well.

Perinatal bereavement counselling

The literature on counselling in the event of perinatal death is not large, but provides useful insights into important issues.

The counsellor

GINNIE: I don't think just one person should do all [the counselling] though. A sister was employed in – Maternity Hospital and she was the counselling sister and it was too much for one person. It needs two to share because you are only human too. You're going to get distressed.

Like midwife Ginnie in my study, Herkes (2002) identifies the need for emotional support in her role as a bereavement counsellor in a maternity unit. The support may be provided by a psychologist, or mutual support may be appropriate if there are two or more colleagues. Herkes describes her role in terms of taking over from the family to provide support when they 'emotionally withdraw' and encourage the couple to 'move on with their life and put the experience behind them' (2002: 135). Herkes's counselling role was built up gradually alongside her formal counselling education from being a labour ward midwife. Eventually, funding from the Child Bereavement Trust permitted Herkes to assume a full-time counselling role. This service is available to parents bereaved in the maternity unit and the neonatal unit, and parents of babies who die due to SIDS up to twelve months.

The majority (60 per cent) of Herkes's referrals are self-referrals, with the remainder being from the full range of caring professions. Most of her referrals are made while the woman is in the maternity unit and there is a quick fall-off with the return home. In support of her contention that she takes over as the family withdraws, there is then a gradual increase in referrals up to six months after the bereavement (2002: 137). Herkes's initial contract with the parent(s) is for six weekly sessions, each lasting for one hour. While 43 per cent of clients complete these six sessions and then end their contact with her, 22 per cent do not complete the six sessions. The remaining 35 per cent of clients may continue being counselled, to the extent of some attending for more than eighteen sessions. The people who attend are predominantly women (55 per cent) who are counselled without their partner. Of the total number of sessions, 29 per cent are for couples attending together. This observation, together with the fact that only 4 per cent of the sessions are for men by themselves, may indicate the different nature of the man's reaction to loss. Unfortunately, although Herkes provides details of who attends, there is no evaluation of the effectiveness of this service in meeting the aims, which she describes as to 'facilitate parents in their grief work' (2002: 137).

The midwife in clinical practice

The relevance of counselling skills to midwives whose job description includes providing support is clear. For three reasons we must question whether these skills are appropriate for other midwives, that is those in clinical practice. First, Burnard and Morrison (1991) indicate the difficulty of using a reflective, client-centred approach in the clinical setting which exerts a number of other, possibly more immediate, demands. Second, much of the work already mentioned emphasises the structured nature of the counselling relationship which may conflict with the somewhat less than structured clinical workload. Third, counselling is not possible while the bereaved person is still in 'a state of numbness or shock', so counselling is unlikely to begin until about a week after the funeral (Worden, 2003).

Although bereavement counselling may not be appropriate during the few hours or days that the grieving mother spends with us in the maternity area, the approaches and skills used in counselling are certainly likely to be helpful. Using the hospital-oriented approach prevalent in the USA, Davis *et al.* (1988) describe the emotional support which is offered on a less than ideal short-term basis. These authors list some practical interventions which are likely to prove helpful:

- encouraging acknowledgement of the birth and death of the baby
- validating feelings of loss and despair
- educating about grief
- giving information about choices available.

Davis *et al.* go on to consider how staff are able to meet the mother's emotional needs. It is essential, also, to cope with the inevitable feelings of failure among staff, which we must acknowledge to be able to help the mother. Taking time to listen to the mother's sad and angry outbursts shows her that these feelings are acceptable and that her isolation is not complete. Anger directed at staff, us or our colleagues may be difficult to accept, but defensiveness may be defused by remembering that her or their anger is unfocused, rather than specific. Our fear of not knowing what to say may make us anxious when in this mother's presence, but remembering the value of listening may reduce anxiety. Many writers list the unhelpful comments which are best avoided (Lendrum and Syme, 1992). It may be helpful to a less-confident or less-experienced staff member to know that she can open the conversation by saying briefly how she feels about the woman's loss. This opening shows the woman that the knowledge is shared and gives her permission, should she want to, to discuss it.

In a UK setting, Kohner and Henley (1992) emphasise the importance of the care of the bereaved mother in the community. The value of the midwife's visits goes far beyond the assessment of the mother's physical condition and provides another opportunity for her to ask questions and talk about her loss. Through a detailed knowledge of the locality in which she practises, the midwife should also be able to help the mother to make contact with a self-help group. Because the surviving child or children are likely to be around when she visits, the midwife is also able to help the parents support their adjustment to the family's loss.

Discussion and summary

A problem raised by the informants in my study, and which is hardly mentioned in the literature, is the extent to which other staff and possibly the mother may 'miss out' if the counselling role is assumed by one person:

RUBY: I don't know if there should be someone specifically in the unit, to help give these mums guidance. I think it's something we've all got to learn to do . . . if you designate one person, you will be left with that person and no one else would bother with them.

NANCY: They're all counselled. The trouble is that it seems to me that most of them are counselled by nursing officers. They do the actual arrangements or speaking to them, counselling the choices about what they intend to do with the baby, whether they want the hospital to bury the baby or whether they want to make their own funeral arrangements.

The risk of misgivings among other staff is mentioned by Druery (1992) in her role as a bereavement support midwife. She avoids confrontation by not usurping other midwives' roles, offering only support and advice to the midwife and by guiding less-experienced practitioners through the paperwork.

Although the structured approach to counselling which I have described here may have limited relevance to the midwife in the maternity unit, the importance of counselling skills in her practice becomes apparent when we consider her twenty-four-hour presence. Davis *et al.* (1988) emphasise that we must be available to be with the mother when she feels she is ready to talk. Unlike the counselling model, this may not be at a pre-determined time, but may be in the small hours when she is at her lowest ebb and other staff are off duty. It is at this time that the midwife is able to listen and use her 'way of being' to help and support the mother (see page 60). Although Worden (2003) indicates that the time when midwives are in contact with the mother may be too early for counselling, midwives are ideally suited to help the mother to recognise and accept her feelings before her formal counselling (if any) begins.

The role of the bereavement counsellor in the maternity area may be questioned, but her existence is widely regarded as valuable in at least two settings. The first is when grieving has been identified as likely to become pathological such as where the mother lacks support from her family and friends and where she has a poor relationship with her partner. The second highly valued contribution of the bereavement counsellor is her input into the introduction of students and midwives to death education.

In this chapter I have considered what bereavement counselling involves, its place in the maternity area and the extent to which it is appropriate for use by midwives. The role of the counsellor has been shown to be similar to that of the midwife, in that the midwife is 'with woman' throughout her experience of childbearing, while the counsellor uses her 'way of being' to help resolve grief. It may be for these reasons that this form of care is so popular among midwives and other maternity carers.

Of greater significance, though, are the serious concerns raised by the systematic reviews of the research evidence on bereavement counselling. In general, counselling and bereavement counselling have been shown to be almost invariably ineffective. To this general picture it is necessary to add the conclusion of Chambers and Chan, which is based on their systematic review of support after perinatal death. These researchers conclude that strong evidence is lacking 'to indicate that routinely offered support, either standard nursing and social support or specialist psychological counselling, has any effect in preventing or reducing pathological grieving and/or long term psychosocial morbidity' (2004). There is obviously a lack of evidence for its benefits and, hence, there is a potential for harm. It is necessary to question, therefore, why resources are being allocated to this questionable activity, rather than to the research to assess its value.

7   Family grief

When contemplating the effects of grief in a family, the concept of 'Gestalt' is helpful. Defined as 'the whole is greater than the sum of the parts' (Drever, 1964), in this context this word implies both the extent and the interdependence of the family components. Family interdependence may not always be easily apparent and as a result the diverse effects of one event, such as a loss, may not be obvious. However, because individual family members are affected by loss, the family system is involved and, hence, all members are affected. Through the interaction of the members and their frequent adjustment and readjustment of roles, however, family homeostasis is ordinarily maintained.

Having emphasised the integrity of the functioning of the family system, in order to examine the differing perceptions and effects of loss, I now find it necessary to separate out the various family members. This is to permit an examination of the differing reactions. As far as possible in thinking about family grief, I focus on the effects of perinatal loss. Where specifically relevant authoritative literature is lacking, though, I draw on more general material, such as that relating to the loss of an older person.

Family

The term 'family' is open to a variety of interpretations, depending largely on the cultural context. All too often in the UK the term is used synonymously with 'nuclear family'. I use the word 'family', though, in its widest sense to include not only those related through blood and marriage or cohabitation, but also foster, adoptive and step-relations. I include also those unrelated adult people who in the past have been (and sometimes still are) honoured with the title 'uncle' or 'aunt' (Baggaley, 1993).

The family as a system

In order to understand the effects of loss on the family, systems theory is useful. This approach is able to take account of dormant or possibly suppressed family characteristics, such as cultural and religious beliefs, ageist and sexist attitudes and status. Group responses may resurface together with inter-generational fictions (Howarth and Leaman, 2001). The systems approach defines the family, first, in terms of being a unit whose interacting parts operate within certain defined boundaries, such as those I have mentioned above. Second, the interaction of the parts is characterised by varying degrees of openness in communication; a family system which adopts a more closed communicative style is typically less flexible to changes in the external environment as well as being less sensitive to the needs of its individual members. Third, as well as physical and other boundaries, the family system operates within its own framework of rules, which may be implicit or explicit. This framework serves to determine the roles of family members within the family system and to maintain, through constant minor readjustments, the homeostasis of the system (Howarth and Leaman, 2001).

Clearly, the death of one of its members seriously threatens the homeostasis of the system. The degree of threat varies according to features of both the family and the death. These features include, first, the timing of the death in the family life cycle, second, the nature of the death, third, the degree of openness within the family and, fourth, the role of the family member who has died. The re-establishment of family equilibrium will follow realignment of roles and reassignment of responsibilities. This realignment constitutes a threat, first, to family stability and, second, to those most closely involved because at this time they are vulnerable and in a weak negotiating position. The factors which further inhibit family coping with loss are categorised by Cook and Oltjenbruns (1989). There may be situational stressors, such as unemployment, which may be cumulative and the effects of which are moderated by the strength of family resources. Family coping may be additionally facilitated by the family's interpretation of the event, in that finding a meaning for the loss renders it more manageable.

Communication within the family

There is a tendency for more responsible members of the family to 'protect' others from the effects of an unpleasant event by limiting communication. This means that in their effort to protect the less involved family members by not discussing the loss, the main actors do not talk about it. This scenario carries dangers both to the protectors, who may not allow themselves to grieve appropriately, and to the protected, who are prevented from experiencing a healthy mourning. Thus, parents may seek to protect their surviving children in this way, to the benefit of neither (see Appendix 2).

The degree of openness of communication within the system is a family characteristic which affects their ability to grieve a lost child. Denial of the loss may feature prominently. The closed family's behaviour may appear bizarre to outsiders, because it responds in ways which have been learned from earlier, but possibly dissimilar, experiences. Thus, the inability of the closed family to accept and share new influences and experiences will limit its coping ability. The family conspiracy of silence (see Appendix 2) which may develop following the death of a child may be attributable to shared guilt. The guilty and unrealistic beliefs about individual personal responsibility for the death are common to all family members, who are united only in their inability to articulate their pain.

Family communication in a hospice setting was the focus of a research project by Lugton (1989). She drew on Glaser and Strauss's account of open and closed awareness among dying people and those near to them (1965). Their original research showed the ease of communication when open awareness operated and all involved knew the terminal nature of the illness. In closed awareness, though, those involved were unable to admit the significance of the illness. Lugton identified varying shades of communication between open and closed awareness in her study. Although her interviewees expressed understanding of the prognosis, the extent to which this understanding was shared within the family varied hugely. Those families in which awareness was open were able to negotiate new roles during the illness, thus preparing themselves for the subsequent major reassignment of roles. Lugton identified the disquiet within families who used closed awareness. Although this research was undertaken in a hospice for adults, there is no reason to suspect that these variable communication patterns do not feature in childbearing loss.

Expectations and perceptions

After looking at social support for widows, Gorer (1965) concluded that the perception of a deficit between expected and experienced support impedes grieving. Since then, the unhelpful nature of interactions has been implicated as responsible, on the grounds that grieving widows who reported few or no unhelpful interactions adjusted better. The reverse was true for widows who perceived more frequent unhelpful activities. The accuracy of these widows' perceptions and the reality of their expectations may be questioned, but it is necessary to accept that the perception of unhelpfulness impairs grieving. In her study, Littlewood (1992) identified four factors perceived as unhelpful and which operated in this way to impede grieving:

1   reduced availability of/access to support
2   family disputes over who is the chief mourner
3   non-acknowledgement of the relationship between the dead person and the bereaved person
4   uncertain social position of the helper.

Parents mourning the loss of a baby may find themselves similarly disappointed by those close to them. They grieve for the baby in whom they had invested hopes and expectations and whom they were coming to know. That their close family are less able to share their loss because they have not been privy to their fantasies may deprive the parents of the support they anticipated. Clearly, this discrepancy between expectations and perceptions may lead to conflict.

Fathers

The role of the father in the family is rightly beginning to attract the attention which it deserves, although the father's actions may not always match expectations (Mander, 2004a). This observation applies as much to childbearing and childrearing loss as to other areas of family activity.

The loss of a viable baby

An important example of a study into the father's experience was undertaken in Sweden as part of a large epidemiological survey of care in the event of perinatal loss (Samuelsson *et al.*, 2001). The researchers were able to undertake qualitative interviews with eleven fathers whose babies had died *in utero* between the twenty-ninth and forty-second weeks of pregnancy. The father's profound sorrow emerges clearly in this work. Although many of the fathers had some suspicion that the baby's condition was not good, they were still severely distressed when told that the baby was dead. The father's immediate concern, however, was to protect his partner. He thought that he should protect her from the pain of labour and that this would be best achieved by a caesarean. The father was accepting, though, when told that this was not necessarily the best course of action.

The lapse of time between being told of the baby's demise and the onset of labour seems to have been highly valued. Whether this time is best spent in the couple's own home or in the relatively protected environment of the maternity unit remains uncertain. Significantly, Samuelsson and colleagues found the father to be disappointed in the information given by staff. This applied, first, on the grounds that he was not included in conversations between members of staff and his partner. Second, he felt that the staff tended to resort to technical jargon which he found incomprehensible. For these men, going home without a baby and returning to work were major hurdles.

Samuelsson and colleagues (2001) were able to draw some comparisons between the man's experience of loss and that of the mother. The differences in the couple's experience of loss led to different coping techniques and, hence, to an improvement in their respect for each other. Sometimes, though, different needs and reactions could lead to unfortunate misunderstandings. The relationship then appears to have become fraught, as both partners sought to avoid aggravating the other's hurt.

These researchers identified the man's wish to locate another man with whom he could share his sorrow. This was especially important in view of men's stereotypical difficulty in 'opening up'. The researchers recognised the 'special fellowship' (2001: 128) which grew up between the fathers in this study. Unfortunately, the reader is not provided with any information about how this fellowship was initiated or how it operated.

The men considered that the taking of mementoes, such as photographs, a lock of hair or a footprint, was later found to be 'invaluable' (2001: 128). They considered that these mementoes should always be taken by staff, even when the mementoes are not wanted by the parents. This recommendation is quite disconcerting, because it raises a host of difficult ethical issues relating to parental autonomy.

As in the research by McCreight (2004) in Northern Ireland, the traditional perception of the father's role as being to protect and to support his partner emerges very clearly from this study. In spite of this, the Swedish researchers indicate that the father's most important wish is for his needs as a bereaved parent to be recognised by those nearby. While these recommendations are clearly eminently reasonable, they may also appear to be contradictory. It may be that the potentially conflicting nature of this father's aspirations may prove particularly taxing for staff. This difficulty may be ameliorated by another important finding of this study, though, which is the father's preparedness to recognise and to articulate his own needs.

The loss of a baby who is miscarried

Miscarriage is one of those topics which serve to throw into sharp relief a number of important issues relating to childbearing loss. This may be because of its relative frequency (Oakley *et al.*, 1990) yet its unexpectedness, as well as its often 'unseen' nature. These factors serve to reduce the significance of miscarriage to many lay people and to many care providers. This insignificance, in turn, is only likely to aggravate the emotional pain of the couple experiencing it.

The severity of emotional reactions to miscarriage was studied by Beutel and colleagues (1996). This study involved a longitudinal assessment to measure the similarities and differences between the reactions of the woman and of the man. These researchers' four hypotheses focused around men grieving less, expressing their grief less, being less attached to the baby and being instrumental in the woman's psychological recovery. The data generally supported the first three hypotheses. The fourth, however, was less straightforward. The women in the study reported that they found that their menfolk were initially supportive and reassuring. After about six months, though, the women were found to be dissatisfied with the level of support provided by their partners and this was found to be associated with a marked increase in 'marital' conflict. These findings are comparable to those of a study in Queensland on perinatal loss (Vance *et al.*, 2002; see page 41).

An attempt to describe the man's perspective on the experience of his partner's early miscarriage was made by Fiona Murphy (1998). She sought to ascertain whether the traditional view of the man endeavouring to be strong for his partner was an accurate reflection of reality in this situation of loss. As with much of the research on men and childbearing (Mander, 2004a), she encountered immense difficulties in locating even a small sample of men for her phenomenological study. After making two false starts, a 'snowball' technique was eventually used to recruit the five men who acted as her informants.

Murphy found that the stereotypical masculine aspiration of 'being strong' was supported by the data which she collected. Additionally, she identified a tendency among the men to blame the hospital personnel for the unpleasantness of the experience of miscarriage. This blame was applied most especially to the perceived mishandling of the breaking of the bad news of the fetal demise. Murphy was able to describe the coping strategies which the man would seek to employ, such as finding distractions, forgetting, and trying to carry on as normal. This research showed that, to the man, recognising the reality of the baby is crucial to his ability to function sympathetically in the event of miscarriage. The obvious corollary is that this recognition is only possible if he has 'seen' the baby during an ultrasound scan. In terms of the implications of her findings, Murphy suggests that better follow-up services should be provided after a miscarriage. Unfortunately, while regretting nurses' insignificant input into this man's care, she does not indicate who would be the best person to provide this follow-up.

Two researchers in England who have also focused on the male partner's experience at the time of miscarriage are Puddifoot and Johnson. In their 1999 publication, these researchers report the findings of a study applying the Perinatal Grief Scale (PGS) to a sample of 323 men. This quantitative study involved collecting data within eight weeks of the miscarriage. These researchers report the widespread assumption that the father is impervious to the pain of loss. Their data, however, serve to contradict this assumption by finding that the grief levels measured in the men were similar to those of women. This study went on to show that there is a strong and positive correlation between the depth of the man's grief and both the duration of the pregnancy and his having seen the ultrasound scan. This latter point resonates with the findings of Fiona Murphy in the context of early miscarriage (see page 41).

Following the data produced by the PGS, Puddifoot and Johnson discuss their observation that involvement in this research project may have served as a cathartic experience for the man who was grieving. This observation is interesting, especially in view of the obvious enthusiasm of the men to be involved in this study. Whereas Fiona Murphy (1998) recounted her serious difficulty in recruiting even five men respondents, in the other research John Puddifoot and Martin Johnson were able to recruit 323 men. These researchers regret that the response rate to the distribution of their research packs was *only* 56 per cent. The reader is only able to surmise why this team of researchers was successful in their recruitment, where others failed so abysmally.

In another publication by Puddifoot and Johnson (1997), they report the qualitative findings of their study undertaken in the north of England. By way of endorsement of my last observation, these researchers report having been in a position to randomly select twenty men from among forty-two volunteers to be interviewed. These researchers were told of a culture of non-communication of the man with his male peers. This inability to share his experiences applied even to the men who had gone through a similar loss as recently as two weeks earlier.

The men reported that they found they were being forced to subscribe to a culture in which men are regarded as strong and showing their feelings of sorrow is not permitted. The expression of grief is widely viewed as a form of self-indulgence. Interestingly, it is not only men who enforced acqui-escence to this cultural norm. One grieving father told of being reprimanded by his own mother when, on finding him tearful, he reported her having said: 'that I was being selfish and had to pull myself together before I upset [my partner]' (1997: 839). In terms of communication with his partner, the man's views varied between two extremes. On the one hand the man was silent, through his fear of saying the wrong thing and causing further upset. On the other hand the man was silent because he considered that the couples' shared feelings were sufficiently eloquent, for their feelings to be beyond words and that there was no need to resort to speech. Uncertainty remains, though, of whether the grief-stricken woman partner would be in a suitably perceptive frame of mind to be able to distinguish between these two extremes.

Serious questions were raised by Puddifoot and Johnson about the legit-imacy or illegitimacy of the man's feelings of sorrow. These researchers suggest that, because of the man's perception that the demonstration of grief is not appropriate for a man in the event of a miscarriage, these men were effectively in denial of their feelings. The men resorted to justifying their lack of grief by regarding the miscarried baby as having been something other than either a 'real' or a 'proper' baby (1997: 840). A distinct element of blame was bound up with these forms of justification, in which the woman was perceived as over-reacting to the miscarriage: 'She just likes making a fuss' (1997: 840). 'She talks about it as if we had actually lost a baby, but we haven't because it had never been born alive' (1997: 840). The men's justifica-tion of the loss by miscarriage tended towards the traditional forms of rationalisation to the effect that this loss was 'Nature's way' (of disposing of a less than perfect baby) (1997: 842). This element of blame was even more overt for some of the men. One man, jealous of his wife's premarital sexual experience, suggested that these activities were responsible for the miscar-riage. Another blamed her active social life: 'She did keep going to the club and who knows what they do on their Friday nights out?' (1997: 842). 'Well, her smoking won't have helped, would it?' (1997: 842). 'Look we do our bit right, then it's up to them, isn't it?' (1997: 842). Some of the men also reported some degree of self-blame. This sometimes took the form of an inability to correct a situation that was going seriously wrong, which was perceived as a significant threat: 'I stood like a lemming not knowing what to do . . . just like a little boy who can't find his mummy' (1997: 841). Such feelings of infantile regression were clearly a threat to the man's self-esteem, as was the risk that he might lose his partner's high regard: 'I'm sure that I will have lost some respect in her eyes now, and rightly so' (1997: 841). For some of the men, the feelings aroused in them by the miscarriage were even more profound. Questions emerged about the meaning or pointlessness of life and the fundamental threat exerted by a loss such as this.

Puddifoot and Johnson summarise their findings in terms of the men's 'unfinished business' which is left over from their own and their partners' past experiences. Some of these relate to childhood, whereas other left-over experiences are more recent. These researchers regret the man's inability to find a role in the event of a miscarriage, which is generally defined as a 'female event'. Puddifoot and Johnson conclude that the man is effectively in what they term a 'double bind'. This amounts to the man feeling that anything which he does will inevitably aggravate the unhappy situation. So his solution is to do nothing. Unfortunately for him, this has the effect of aggravating the situation, because it causes him to appear to be uncaring. The researchers' analysis, however, fails to take account of the effect of the time warp in which women have become able to talk more openly about unhappy events such as miscarriage. Men, however, have either excluded themselves or have been excluded from these conversations. According to Puddifoot and Johnson, some men are suffering from serious emotional pain as a consequence.

Couples

We tend to assume that babies are always born into relationships like those which we knew as children and which involve people of opposite sexes. This is not necessarily so. In this section particularly we must bear in mind that, though I tend to refer to heterosexual couples because they have been studied, my observations are likely to apply equally to lesbian, and possibly gay, couples. Similarly, I focus on couples, but we should also remember the unsupported mother who may need to grieve not only the loss of her baby, but also the loss of her relationship with her baby's father.

It may be assumed that the father's grief corresponds qualitatively and quantitatively with the mother's. Research findings help to clarify this issue.

Mother/father differences in grieving

On the basis of their work with widows, Stroebe and Stroebe (1987) identified the variation between individuals in the duration and progress of grieving, as well as people's tendency to oscillate and hesitate between stages. These observations have led to the dual process theory of grieving (see page 7). Dual process involves the person's grief or mourning behaviour moving between the passive 'feminine' inactivity and the stereotypically 'masculine' pursuit of resolution.

The traditional view of the gendered nature of grief has recently been subjected to a certain degree of reinterpretation (Stroebe and Schut, 1995). Thompson (1997) reflects on the traditional assumptions about masculine grieving being characterised by 'emotional inexpressiveness' (1997: 77). He attributes these assumptions, not to innate traits in men, but to their more active coping style of mourning. In Western society such activity may not actually be recognised as mourning. Because of his activity and others' non-recognition of his grieving and mourning the man may be perceived as a problem by those who might be able to offer him help. This is likely to be associated with difficult relationships with would-be helpers and the non-availability of support when he seeks it (Thompson, 1997: 82).

Perhaps because the mother is invariably present at the birth, there is a tendency to use and accept her view of the experience. Whether this is appropriate when thinking about fathers' reactions is questionable. For this reason I focus here on research which has deliberately sought a balanced view of the couple's experience. An additional reason for the difficulty in interpreting the material on fathers' grieving (Littlewood, 1992) is that men may under-report or fail to acknowledge the disruption which they experience. As Dyregrov (1991) states in the context of young boys, the difficulty which they encounter in articulating their grief may continue into adult life as difficulty in even recognising its existence.

Dissynchrony and asymmetry

JOSIE: It may take them a wee while to accept it. You may have one partner accepting it and the other one not.

Midwife Josie in my study recognised the potential for variation in grieving. The reason why grieving and coping styles assume such significance in the context of perinatal death is associated with the incorrect assumption, mentioned already, that we all grieve similarly. Unfortunately, each parent may assume that, because they have lost the same baby, their grief will manifest itself similarly. They may have difficulty in realising that their coping mechanisms, their hopes and expectations for their baby and their relationship with that baby may not have been identical. In two parents of different sexes the grieving of each is likely to progress in different ways and at different rates. Each parent may assume that, because their partner is not grieving as they are, then they are not grieving appropriately. Typically, the mother is still overtly grieving while the father is returning to work.

The differences in grieving may be in terms of, first, dissimilar gender-determined manifestations, second, dissynchrony, meaning that their emotional roller-coasters are poorly aligned and, third, asymmetry or incompatibility in their grief responses (Singg, 2003: 885).

A large longitudinal study was undertaken in Queensland, Australia by Vance and colleagues (2002) to measure 'distress' among couples bereaved by stillbirth, neonatal death or sudden infant death syndrome (SIDS). 'Distress' was measured by quantitative instruments which focused on anxiety, depression and alcohol intake. According to Boyle, a large majority of the sample in the same study comprised parents bereaved by stillbirth or neonatal death (207 respondents out of 259: 80 per cent) (1997: 62). Yet again, the common problem of accessing and retaining a suitably large sample of men proved challenging. These researchers found that the couple's different expectations of each other's grief were important in the development of their relationship. The fathers were found to be quite accepting of the woman's severe distress and recognised the significance of her loss. The woman, on the other hand, tended to be unhappy when she perceived the man to be less distressed than she was. In this unfortunate situation, the relationship was found to be likely to begin to deteriorate. This incongruity or asymmetry of the couple's grieving is apparent in the respondents' distress scores. The women's distress declined gradually and consistently over the thirty-month period of data collection. This contrasts with the men's, albeit lower, scores, which peaked at thirty months.

With two parents in a highly sensitive and vulnerable state the potential for conflict is massive. One may blame the other for being uncaring while the other makes accusations of wallowing in grief. Each may be unable or unwilling to appreciate the other's viewpoint, if it has been articulated. As a result, each may wonder whether the other's loving feelings towards them have changed. They may feel that they are alone in their grief. In the absence of effective communication, each partner will continue to think badly of the other. Singg (2003) discusses one route of communication with which this couple may have particular difficulty; this is their sexual relationship (see Chapter 13).

Changes in the relationship

Inevitably, as the two individuals who make up the couple will be changed by their experience of loss, so their relationship will undergo changes. The nature of these changes is a source of contention as some writers foretell serious adverse consequences in the form of break-up (Singg, 2003). Although a high divorce rate among bereaved parents is mentioned, it is difficult to locate supporting evidence. A large survey was undertaken in the USA by a market research organisation (NFO Research Inc.), focusing on the parental experience following the loss of a child from miscarriage to maturity (TCF, 2002). After a small volunteer response, 304 women and 290 men were interviewed by telephone. As usual the researchers were unable to contact an equal sample of fathers. The researchers appeared to be reassured by the fact that 72 per cent of the parents who were married at the time of the death remained married to the same spouse.

In the event of the relationship becoming difficult following the loss of a baby, secondary losses, such as the loss of family unity, may follow the death which constituted the primary loss. The secondary loss may be real, or it may be symbolic, such as the loss of some part of oneself. As well as secondary losses, though, it is not impossible that some secondary gains may eventually present themselves.

Grandparents

More appropriate research attention to grandparents and greatgrandparents is now beginning to correct their traditional sentimentalisation (Gelles, 1995). This development may be due to demographic changes, which mean that grandparents are relatively young and healthy, as well as the increasing fragility of 'marital' relationships requiring greater family support. Recognition of the benefits of grandparental involvement in childrearing is also comparatively recent, which may be associated with demographic changes as well as the modification of ageist attitudes. Their involvement may comprise emotional support or information-giving or even financial support.

Their input is unique among non-parents, which may be explained by their 'vested interest in the development of the grandchild' (Brubaker, 1987: 71). Grandparents' contribution to childrearing varies according to whether they are maternal or paternal family and grandmothers or grandfathers; in both, the former are invariably more involved (Smith, 1991). Additional factors which affect grandparental involvement relate to their age, their employment, their social class, their geographical location, their ethnic origin, whether they are institutionalised, whether they are blood relations and their personality (Hurme, 1991). Cunningham-Burley's (1984) research showed the grandparents' prevalent desire that their involvement in childrearing should comprise a positive but non-interfering role.

In the same way as the father's role is sometimes assumed to be only to support the mother, the grandparents may be perceived as having no involvement in the process of loss other than to support the parents (McHaffie, 1991). Research literature does not support this view.

Loss of future

The significance of the new baby to the grandparents derives from her symbolic representation of the future, and if the baby is lost they perceive a threat to the continuity of the family and life generally (Long, 1992). In certain ways grandparents consider that, because they have invested their hopes and expectations in this baby, she belongs to them as well as to the parents. Thus, their grief is aggravated.

Inability to help own child

Their inability to compensate their child for her loss of her baby or to protect their child from her grief is a source of misery to grandparents (TCF, 2003). Now that she has proved herself adult in the most obvious way, they are no longer able to fulfil their parental role and feel they have become marginalised and superfluous. Grandparents may be unaware of the significance which their children attach to their emotional support at difficult times (Smith, 1991; McHaffie, 1991).

Survivor guilt

The untimeliness of perinatal death reminds grandparents and greatgrandparents that as they are nearer the end of their life-span it is they, not the new baby, who should die. The grandparents' grief is compounded by the feeling of inappropriateness of the loss of the young, when the old survive. These feelings are likely to be aggravated by their non-recognition by others (TCF, 2003).

Grandparenting AIDS orphans

Children whose parents die of AIDS may be 'fortunate' enough to be raised by their grandparents (Nord, 1997: 168). Inevitably, though, both children and grandparents will continue to face a number of challenges. These include the loss of a generation in the family and the effect on the relationship of the age difference between the child and her surrogate parents.

Grandparents' grieving

In her study of family support and bereavement, Kowalski (1987) interviewed grandparents in five families. Just as others have noted the reluctance of fathers to cry, the grandfathers were factual and unemotional, whereas the grandmothers were more open in sharing their emotions. The maternal grandmothers' primary concern was the welfare of their daughters; grief at the loss of their grandchild was secondary. As observed already, paternal grandparents were less intensely involved. Grandparents regretted being unable to protect their child from grief, but failed to relate such feelings to the grief of the parents about losing 'their' child.

The reality of the dead baby was hard for grandparents to accept. Kowalski found that the grief of some of the grandmothers related not to the recently lost baby, but to other losses, earlier in their lives. The difficulty of grandmothers' grieving has also been identified elsewhere. Only grandmothers who have been the primary caregiver of the dead child really grieve. Other grandmothers' grief relates to the loss of another, somewhere in the past. It may be that we should provide support for those who grieve irrespective of the source of their grief and not limit support only to the current loss.

Loss in multiple pregnancy

The demands and joys of twins are many, especially if the conception follows a period of infertility. The increasing availability of assisted reproduction techniques (ART) is thought to be responsible for the marked increase in the twinning rate and, even more, the higher-order multiple births (Petterson *et al.*, 1998). Alongside this potentially good news, we must remember that multiple pregnancy and birth carries many risks for both the woman and her babies. This is reflected in the estimate that '15% of multiples grow up as singleton survivors' (Swanson *et al.*, 2002: 156). For the sake of convenience, I refer to all multiple births here as twins.

The loss of a twin may occur at various times and in different ways. Spontaneous loss during pregnancy may be recognised or it may be unknown. The 'vanishing twin' (see page 41) is now more likely to be recognised due to the frequent use of ultrasound. Without this investigation the presence of a *'fetus papyraceous'* would only be recognised after the birth.

Because of the increased incidence of higher-order multiples with ART or because of an abnormality in a baby, interventions for 'partial' termination may be possible in the first trimester. These techniques may be known as 'selective feticide', 'selective birth' or 'selective reduction' (Price, 1992: 109; Evans *et al.*, 1998). The lack of research into the experience of the woman or couple undergoing these procedures indicates that these interventions are yet another example of medical technology having outstripped the legal and human understanding which they require.

The loss of one of the babies later in pregnancy or neonatally may be due to twin transfusion syndrome. The high level of neonatal deaths among twins may be associated with their likely prematurity, the risk of one or both suffering some degree of intra-uterine growth retardation or their increased likelihood of some congenital abnormality (Petterson *et al.*, 1998).

The loss of a twin, or one or more of the babies if a higher multiple, has some aspects in common with loss of a singleton baby, but there is a 'particular sorrow' (McHaffie, 2001: 45).

Gratitude

The assumption may be made that the parents should be so grateful to have one healthy baby that they should not need to grieve the loss of the one who died (Bryan, 1999). This assumption may manifest itself in potentially hurtful comments: 'When we were told he would die, they told us very quickly and then the consultant jumped quickly to saying that I had another baby (his twin)' (bereaved mother, in Redshaw *et al.*, 1996: 181). Such misunderstanding may hinder the parents' grieving. The presence of a living twin has been shown to in no way ameliorate the impact of the parents' loss. Rather than having an easier time, the parents of twins when one dies may actually find more difficulty in grieving for one baby and forming a relationship with another simultaneously.

The problem of grieving one baby

The danger of not grieving the loss of one twin lies in the inevitable eventual manifestation of the grief, possibly in a severely pathological form. The difficulty of grieving one baby and simultaneously beginning a new relationship with another is discussed in Chapter 13. The parents face problems in coping with these contradictory psychological processes simultaneously. There is the danger that the dead baby may be dismissed as a mere fantasy; but this can only be a temporary dismissal, with the grieving being nothing more than delayed, appearing later as one of the syndromes of failed mourning. These pathological outcomes may be avoided by ensuring that the family have experienced the reality of the dead baby, and that they have some tangible memories of her.

Blaming the survivor

The family may show their grief at the loss of a twin by blaming the one who survived. While blaming the live baby, the dead twin may be idealised; this 'angel baby' is particularly likely to materialise if the survivor is in any way unwell or badly behaved (Bryan, 1999). To make up to her, the family may then try to overcompensate the survivor.

The lone twin

Regardless of the gestation or age at which the other twin dies, the survivor feels at some level responsible for the death, a form of survivor guilt. This may appear like the separation anxiety seen in older twins. The difficulty of distinguishing self and not-self in infants may persist in twins and causes problems when a twin does not survive. The parents should be open with the survivor about the death of the twin and be prepared to produce photographs of the babies together to establish their separate identities (Bryan, 1999).

The vanishing twin

With the increasing use of ultrasound early in pregnancy, there is increasing awareness of the 'vanishing twin' (Newman, 1998: 112). Possibly because of placental malfunction, one twin does not survive the early months of pregnancy and is reabsorbed or may be found after the birth as a *fetus papyraceous*. Whether to inform the parents of the presence of two babies is a contentious issue, but Bryan (1992) suggests that the family's awareness of the twin may be important.

The loss of twin motherhood

The excitement, joy, social status and magical feelings engendered by twins in our society contrast markedly with the pain of complicated grief. This may be less significant than the loss of self-esteem, even shame, faced by a mother who loses a twin (Bryan, 1999).

Sibling perinatal loss

When a child's unborn or newborn sibling dies, the child faces a wide variety of emotions, which may include personal disappointment, parental sorrow and general disturbance. The emotions which do or do not manifest themselves vary with the age and understanding of the child. As the child grows older and her understanding changes and increases, the meaning of the death also changes from the initial, perhaps guilt-ridden, reaction. Sorrow among parents and other adults means that the child's interpretation of the loss and its current and future significance may be neglected. The consequences are far-reaching, but, with appropriate care, harm may be avoided.

The role of those caring for bereaved parents is not only to help them to grieve for the one who is lost, but also, and perhaps more challengingly, to help them to think of the future for themselves and their family. The care of surviving children is a crucial aspect of care.

In thinking about sibling reactions to perinatal loss, my focus is primarily on young children, particularly of pre-school age. This is because families are currently small with short gaps, so it is young children who are more likely to be affected by perinatal sibling loss. The lack of relevant research-based material requires me to use material about other age-groups and a case-study (Appendix 2).

Children's understanding

Although children are frequently exposed to death, it is almost invariably through television. This medium detaches the viewer from the reality of the event and does not help a child understand this taxing concept; additionally, viewing the same actor in another programme subsequently may carry misleading messages. So how does a child learn the meaning of death?

It is usual to think of a child's understanding of death in terms of the developmental stage which she has achieved. The cognitive framework introduced by Piaget and expanded by Kastenbaum (2000) may seem appropriate, envisaging the child passing through stages featuring concreteness, centration, egocentrism, irreversibility, animism and fantasy to reach transductive reasoning. Hayslip and Hansson (2003) explain these stages in terms of the initial phase of denial which regards death as like a form of sleep. The second stage death is either personalised or externalised and it is not until the third stage that the young person realises the universal, unavoidable and irrevocable nature of death. In small children, concrete thinking predominates and abstractions relating to the location of the dead person may be less than helpful, as one midwife told me:

NANCY: . . . a woman who'd had five miscarriages, her first baby was born alive and he was nine . . . and he asked me if he could see his brothers and sisters because they had been born here but couldn't come home, so he wanted to see them.

The information given to this boy had clearly not taken account of his limited understanding.

The characteristics of death which we all have ultimately to master are non-functionality, universality, causality and personification. A child's view of life as cyclical may prevent her from accepting the immutability of death in that people who die do not come back to life. This may be associated with a child's tendency to think in egocentric, magical terms, which leads her to think that she can bring the baby back to life; but it may also burden her with nagging anxieties about her own responsibility for the baby's death. A child who initially felt ambivalent about the 'arrival of a rival' (Pereira, 2004) may encounter guilt because of her earlier hostile thoughts. Her egocentricity may initiate a guilty cycle of non-communication if her parents are unable to provide factual information (McNeil, 1986).

Because a child may not fully comprehend the implications of the word 'death', her reaction to being given sad news may be quite different from that of an older person. She may not accept the permanence of death, as the concept of future time may not yet be real. Such 'inappropriate' and apparently callous reactions may cause pain to a grieving parent.

The difficulties which a child faces may be addressed in perplexing ways. For example, denial and magical thinking are ways of coping with loss. Such fantasies may become established as part of denial, which serve to retard the grieving process. While we are aware of the fantasies which mothers who have not seen their stillborn babies may harbour, we can only imagine that the fantasies of uninformed children are yet more fearful (see Appendix 2).

The age at which a child's understanding is sufficient for her to be informed of loss is a contentious point (see Appendix 2). Understanding clearly relates to the developmental stage, as already mentioned, but this may be advanced by family and other experience (Howarth and Leaman, 2001). While some authors suggest a specific age at which understanding is achieved, it is difficult to imagine that an even younger child is not aware of the disruption and grief among those near to her, and hence deserves appropriate explanations.

Physical and behavioural responses

An important feature of the groundbreaking research by Dyregrov (1988) was its detailed description of sibling grief in a healthy child population. This researcher followed up seventy-five families who had experienced a perinatal death or early SIDS and had surviving children; there was a respectable 55 per cent response rate to his initial approach. A longitudinal design collected quantitative and qualitative data from parents about the grief of three- to nine-year-olds.

Anxiety was found to be a prominent if short-term feature, which was apparent in the child's sleeping difficulties and concern about parental health. The child constantly sought meaning by questioning the whys and hows of the loss. Repetitive questioning allowed the child to obtain new information and integrate it with old. Many questions were of a concrete nature, relating to the location of heaven, activities in the grave and nourishment. The parents were particularly disturbed by the child's tendency to blame them and show anxiety about their poor caretaking. The child's angry and aggressive responses suggested the existence of affection for the dead child. Although elements of guilt are usually thought to prevail, Dyregrov found little evidence of this.

Behaviourally, Dyregrov identified increasing demands among the grieving children, which were more pronounced in children who had been separated from their parents by being sent to stay with family. Regressive behaviour also features in a child's grief response, including overdependency, separation anxiety, enuresis and social withdrawal.

An issue raised by Dyregrov (1988), which makes the interpretation of his data more difficult, is the close positive correlation between the parental and sibling reactions. It may be that parental grief causes the child to become confused and fearful. The difficulty of separating the child's reaction to the death from the child's reaction to parental grief is aggravated by the tendency of the child to imitate parental behaviour (see Appendix 2). The absence of direct or observational data about the children in Dyregrov's study compounds this problem.

Interventions

On the basis of his research Dyregrov (1988) recommends that the care of grieving children should focus on four areas:

1   **Open and honest communication** – The child should be given an explanation appropriate to her understanding and age, which may be assisted by real-life examples such as the death and burial of a pet or small animal.

    In order to reduce the child's confusion, euphemisms for death should be strenuously avoided. Although the thesaurus lists many alternative words, a child would find difficulty applying them; others would actually cause greater confusion. Examples are 'laid to rest' or 'gone to sleep', which may engender fear of these activities in a child. Similarly, the commonly used euphemism 'lost' may cause yet more confusion. Although adults may find religious observance a solace in grief, complex religious concepts may perplex a small child. A midwife, however, recommended such analogies:

IRENE: I sometimes tell the mother to tell the other children that the new baby was too good for this world and that it has gone to heaven.

An abstract concept, like heaven, presents problems to a toddler.

In order to tell children sad news, there may be difficulty in opening up the topic (see Appendix 2). Questions to probe the child's understanding of the situation may achieve both ends. Dyregrov (1991) recommends that accurate factual information should always be consistently emphasised.

Parents have traditionally tried to protect their children from pain by not informing them of a loss (see Appendix 2). This is merely parental self-protection and in no way benefits the child (Dyregrov, 1988). Ideally, it is parents who give this information, but, unfortunately, they are temporarily, through their own grief, least able to offer it. However, the expression and sharing of sorrow may benefit both parent and child, as when children comfort their grieving parents (Dyregrov, 1988).

2 **Give time for cognitive mastery** – Helping the child's understanding may be time-consuming and painful, but the information needs to be given in packages that the child is able to assimilate. Questioning and openness should be encouraged and may be assisted by more tangible mementoes, such as photographs and items belonging to the baby (see Appendix 2). Visiting the grave is a way of encouraging the child to recognise her loss. Despite cultural opposition to children attending the funeral, Dyregrov found that 35 per cent of his sample had accompanied parents to visit the grave; admittedly, though, this may have been simply for convenience. While sounding incongruous, children are encouraged to work through their grief by play.

3 **Make the loss real** – In Dyregrov's sample almost none of the children had seen their dead sibling, the exceptions being the deaths due to SIDS. In cultures where viewing the body is usual, children are often exempt, but attitudes to children seeing or even holding the dead baby are changing. The child needs to be both prepared for this experience and accompanied by a supportive adult (Dyregrov, 1988, 1991).

Adequate preparation and a specific support person are also essential if, after having been given the choice, the child elects to attend the funeral. Although Dyregrov (1988) considers that attendance is likely to help the child, he stresses that no force or encouragement should be applied. Alternative goodbyes may be arranged if the child decides against the funeral, such as special services or other events.

Perhaps because it is widely used in the UK and because it raises special issues, cremation needs to be mentioned. Dyregrov (1991) suggests that particularly full explanations are essential, as well as suitable follow-up.

Recognising the loss may also be facilitated by parents showing their own feelings openly and by not hiding away mementoes of the dead baby (see Appendix 2).

4   **Stimulate emotional coping** – The practice of 'protecting' a child by removing her from her usual surroundings at a difficult time serves only to increase her separation anxiety (Dyregrov, 1988; see Appendix 2). He found that children who had been separated from their parents became obsessively over-protective towards them.

As well as having a specific adult to accompany a child at sensitive times, a facilitator should be available to help the child to grieve. The school nurse role may encompass this area (Simmons, 1992).

Summary

This chapter has examined some of the wider-ranging effects of perinatal loss. The diversity of the family and the multiplicity of inputs increase its strength and ability to withstand the onslaughts to which it is vulnerable. Despite this, it is apparent that difficulties may arise within families at this time, perhaps associated with all family members being affected, albeit in differing ways, by the death. The extent of threat posed by these difficulties is related to the openness of family communication.

8 Grief in the neonatal unit

When a baby is admitted to the neonatal unit (NNU) it is either because a health problem has been recognised or because there is a real possibility of such a problem arising. Regardless of her diagnosis, the parents of this baby have to adjust to the likelihood of a condition which threatens her health, or even her life (Redshaw *et al.*, 1996). In order to make this adjustment the parents must grieve for the ideal baby or 'inside baby' they expected and have lost (Lewis, 1976, 1979a), before being able to relate to the baby who has been born (see Chapter 4). Thus, even in the absence of death, grief features prominently in the NNU.

A further factor requiring adjustment in these parents is the non-fulfilment of the role which they had anticipated. Ordinarily the mother is able to satisfy her baby's everyday needs, and in doing so she is likely to have the support of midwives, nurses and others. For a mother whose baby has been admitted to the NNU, the situation is reversed and the nurses (including midwives in this chapter) are the primary caregivers. This serves to diminish her self-esteem, by implying that she is incompetent and, hence, 'subsidiary' in the care of her own child (Lupton and Fenwick, 2001).

If the NNU is a large one, it will comprise a Neonatal Intensive Care Unit (NICU), a high-dependency unit (HDU) and a Special Care Baby Unit (SCBU); a NICU is where staff are able to provide more complex life-support systems and, thus, has higher staffing ratios. In this chapter I use the term NNU to include the three levels of care, unless specifically referring to one area. I consider here the care of the family whose baby is at risk of dying in a NNU. Because more intensive care would be appropriate for such a baby, my focus tends more towards that area of the NNU.

Strictly speaking the neonatal period ends twenty-eight days after the birth, but for many babies in the NNU the time since their birth is much greater. They are still at risk, however, of developing health problems which may cause their death. To avoid confusion, I consider here babies who are born alive, but who may die in this setting, rather than those who die at a certain chronological age. I use the term 'newborn' to indicate this less precise meaning.

In many ways, the grief which arises from the death of a newborn is similar to grief at other times; but, as there are certain unique aspects, my focus here is on those features of loss in the NNU which cause it to differ from other forms of loss. I look, first, at the ways in which grieving a newborn is unique and, second, at the help which is available to the bereaved parents. Then I consider decision-making about the continuation or limitation of care in this area and, finally, I look at the setting in which this care is provided and the extent to which the environment may affect caring.

Grieving a death in the NNU

There are many accounts of the unique nature of grieving a newborn. The two major sources, however, appear to complement each other to provide a complete picture of this experience (Redshaw *et al.*, 1996; Benfield *et al.*, 1976). The USA study by Benfield and colleagues comprises a sample of fifty couples and describes authoritatively yet poignantly the feelings of bereaved parents. Redshaw and colleagues surveyed fifty-six NNUs in England, collecting data from staff and parents. Of the nineteen bereaved families in their study, twelve (63 per cent) returned the completed questionnaires, which focused mainly on organisational issues.

Despite the different continents and time, the fact that the babies were of similar size (Table 8.1) suggests that the findings may be comparable.

Benfield and colleagues asked each parent to indicate their measure of grief in seven key areas: feeling sad, loss of appetite, sleeplessness, being more irritable, being preoccupied with the dead baby, feeling guilty about the baby's death and feeling angry. These researchers concluded that grieving a newborn is a highly individual experience and is unrelated to birth weight, age/gestation of the baby at death, degree of parental contact, previous perinatal loss or parental age. Benfield and colleagues used parents' additional comments to draw up a list of concerns which were raised as frequently as items on the questionnaire were ticked.

Anger, directed at both the staff and God, pervaded the experience of a large majority of the parents. It carried with it a significant element of blame, some of which was self-blame, more commonly known as guilt (Singg, 2003). Although these researchers do not detail the source of the parents' guilt, there is a tendency for the mother to analyse all her activities in order to blame those which caused her child's death. An example would be the mother's self-care, which may have been criticised during pregnancy because of smoking or not resting, and thus aggravating her guilt. This guilt-analysis

Table 8.1 Babies' birth weight in two studies

Study	Mean	Range
Benfield *et al.* (1976)	1.994 kg	0.790 kg – 4.080 kg
Redshaw *et al.* (1996)	1.90 kg	0.640 kg – 3.54 kg

may constitute part of grieving, being comparable with the bargaining noted by Kübler-Ross (1970).

Disbelief or unreality was also raised (Benfield *et al.*, 1978), which may relate to the rarity of death of a newborn, or at least to the taboo on mentioning it socially. Alternatively, disbelief may indicate that some degree of denial still persists, as shown by the quote from one mother: 'I keep waiting for the phone to ring, to wake up from my sleep and hear my baby crying.' These researchers were able to describe the 'awkward moments' encountered by the grieving couple. These include the ordinarily innocuous questions such as 'What did you have?' from a casual acquaintance or another mother in the maternity unit. More serious are the incidents attributable to failures in communication in the health care system, such as the respondent whose obstetrician enquired after her baby's health (Benfield *et al.*, 1978). My own experience is that these 'awkward moments' still occur, such as when I was recently admitting a new mother to the postnatal ward, knowing that her baby, having been born at twenty-five weeks, was dying in the NNU. Her obstetric notes had stayed with her baby, so I did not even know the sex of her baby, let alone the details of the birth. My problems were only compounded by my inability to speak her language.

In the USA study, the feelings aroused by the post-mortem (PM) emerged when the parents reported their uncertainty about whether to attend to learn of the result. Downs (2003) discusses some of the reasons for decisions about a PM, including seeking as much information as possible in the hope of preventing a recurrence. Those who decline permission for a PM may have a religious reason. Parental concerns about inappropriate removal of tissue during PM may now have been resolved (DoH, 2003). It may be that parents want their family to 'view the body' to assist their grieving and the anticipated disfigurement would be counterproductive (Chiswick, 2001). Alternatively, they may feel that their baby has gone through enough already without what they see as this final insult. In the research by McHaffie and colleagues this was the most common reason, which was closely followed by the observation that the post-mortem was not necessary because 'the parents had no unanswered questions' (2001: 172).

Concerns about the NNU featured prominently in Redshaw and colleagues' work (1996). It was found that the presence of monitoring and other equipment was a source of anxiety, rather than reassurance, during the crucial first contact between parents and baby. The baby appearing to look like something other than the stereotypical picture of a newborn baby also worried them, as did the noise of the NNU. The bereaved parents were more concerned about problems associated with their communication with staff than parents whose baby survived.

Factors which may make grieving a newborn less difficult

> On a scale of one to ten, when your child dies it's always ten.
>
> (Mother, in McHaffie, 2001: 5)

Although I must assert that grief is never easy, it has been suggested that certain features of the death of a newborn make grieving less difficult. One example is the idea that neonatal death is not as incomprehensible as stillbirth. It may be that the baby's longer period of independent survival correlates with less bewilderment for those nearby. Further, the horror and feeling of overturning of the natural order associated with stillbirth is absent. The parents' grieving is thought to be assisted by their having been able to do the things that parents ordinarily do, such as seeing and holding the live baby. Further, there is a legal requirement for certification of both the birth and the death of a baby who has lived independently, which may also serve to make the death of a newborn more like other deaths and reduce the risk of failed mourning. This view is supported by the suggestion that the greater involvement, and investment, of staff in the care of a dying newborn increases the likelihood of the parents, first, recognising that their baby really lived and, second, being well supported (Littlewood, 1992).

The tendency to regard the death of a newborn as less deserving of grieving than the death of an older person is founded on the societal assumption that less contact with the newborn requires or arouses less grief. This assumption ignores the affection which the mother develops towards the baby before birth. Comparing the ease or difficulty of one form of grief with another is dangerous. Grief is fundamentally individual and there may be other 'baggage' facing the parents which, unknown to us, affects their grieving. We should beware of trivialising or underestimating the significance of any experience of grief. It is necessary to accept that, as has been said of pain, grief 'is what the person experiencing it says it is' (McCaffery, 1979).

The likelihood of the death of a newborn being trivialised was demonstrated by a research project which studied the events and personal interactions which either helped or hindered seven couples' grieving (Helmrath and Steinitz, 1978). As well as confirming the differences in grieving between the mothers and the fathers, these researchers illuminated the extreme isolation of these parents from friends and family. Feelings of guilt were found to predominate. The bereaved parents were distressed by the assumption that the death of a baby was essentially different from the loss of an older child, as evidenced by friends' insensitive comments and unwillingness to mention the baby. Helmrath and Steinitz attribute this unhelpful behaviour to the belief that the baby is replaceable. Others' lack of contact with the baby leads them to feel that grief is misplaced. As a result of these observations, the authors suggest that the bereaved parents should recognise their loss and grieve as they feel necessary.

Factors that may make grieving a newborn more difficult

As I have shown already, others' tendency to underestimate the significance of the death of a newborn in itself constitutes a barrier to grieving. There are a number of other factors which may further impede grieving.

Making contact

The parents' perceptions of the atmosphere of the NNU as a place to begin and to end contact with their newborn was addressed by Redshaw and colleagues. While most of the families were positive about the environment, others found it to be 'hostile', 'depressing' or 'frightening' (1996: 180). These misgivings persisted, in spite of these parents having used the 'quiet room' where they could be with their baby (1996: 180).

The difficulty of the mother being able to make contact with her ill baby is aggravated by the likelihood that she is being cared for in the maternity unit and her child is in the NNU, which may be distant. This problem will be further compounded by her immobility if the birth was by caesarean, which is often trivialised by being referred to as 'caesarean section', or if she has an otherwise incapacitating problem. If the mother and baby are in different hospitals, suggesting geographical distance, other problems may supervene. These may include lack of communication, and perhaps trust, between the staff of different units. It is possible that the mother may be the only way in which the two clinical areas share information and, thus, she will be required to negotiate her way through two very different cultures at a time when all her energy should be focused on her relationship with her baby.

It is necessary to consider the rationale for transferring an ill baby away from her mother soon after birth. The problems of separation are aggravated when the mother has not been given an opportunity to get to know her child (McCabe, 2002). This is less of a problem when the mother gives birth in a conurbation, where transport is easy, but it carries considerable cost and emotional implications in more remote areas. The ideal arrangement is for mother and baby to be transferred together to a maternity unit with the necessary NNU as well as suitable postnatal facilities. This avoids the family being split up between at least three sites. Although neonatal mortality and morbidity have been shown to be reduced by *in utero* transfers, the outcome for the mother may be less than ideal. This has been demonstrated by Bennett and colleagues (2002) who found that the woman's experience of the birth, her health and welfare and even her life may be threatened during these transfers which are intended to be in her baby's interests.

The geographical difficulties associated with the mother still remaining in the maternity unit become particularly acute should her baby die. The mother's non-involvement in arranging her baby's funeral while she is still in hospital may be a deliberate ploy to 'spare' her pain; thus the family and undertakers collude for her presumed welfare. So that the mother's wishes about the funeral will be followed, the funeral may need to be postponed until she is fit to participate. Although it is unusual for a mother to be too unwell to attend the funeral, I have known mothers who have found this difficult. One mother who had a longstanding wound infection appreciated the importance of attending the service and was eventually supported by her family in making the journey. Another mother, a devout Muslim, was prevented by her 'unclean' status from attending, while making a difficult recovery from her caesarean. A service could be arranged in her hospital room for the mother who is too ill to leave the maternity unit.

A bereavement consultant in a NICU, Nichols (1986) attributes many of the grieving problems encountered by parents of dying newborns to discounted grief and negated death. She cites the non-involvement of the mother in the funeral and the equation of 'no contact' with 'no grief' as examples. She recounts some of the hurtful clichés which reflect the negation of newborn death, such as 'You weren't really a mother; why are you acting this way?' The significance of negation is due to it depriving the bereaved parent of social support and inhibiting the progress of grief work.

The potential for an unexpectedly rapid sequence of premature birth and newborn death further serves to impede grieving. As a bereaved parent herself, Nichols (1986) reports that half of the deaths in the NICU where she worked happened within sixty-eight hours of birth. For this reason, the new parents find themselves in a shocked and confused state, to the extent that they feel uncertain whether they are grieving the baby of their prenatal fantasies or a baby who has actually been born. They feel unable to differentiate where their hopes and dreams end and where the reality begins.

Because of this confusion, the parents experience uncertainty about whether to continue to develop their attachment to their ill baby. They are anxious that, in the event of the baby dying, their investment of love and affection will take its toll in grief. Their indecisiveness aggravates their guilt at not feeling an overwhelming surge of love for their baby. It may be that the parents' uncertainty about forming a relationship with their baby is linked to the need to first prepare themselves for the possible loss of their child, that is, the need for anticipatory grieving.

Anticipatory grieving

The benefits and hazards of anticipatory grieving have been debated since Lindemann first introduced the term in 1944. If we view anticipatory grieving prospectively, we see the benefits to the bereaved person, in terms of the gentle modification of grief when death does come, allowing equilibrium to be regained more easily (Howarth and Leaman, 2001). Alternatively, looking at it retrospectively, the damage to the relationship is all too easily apparent if the dying person does not succumb. It is disconcertingly easy to confuse anticipatory grieving with forewarning of loss. Whereas forewarning is simply that, anticipatory grieving comprises a complex interplay of psychological, physical and social factors which serve to make it crucially different from post-mortem grief. The psychological differences involve the intensification of certain aspects and the relief of others; so the depth of guilt, despondency and anger vary hugely. The non-recognition of anticipatory grieving reduces the social interactions and social support to the bereaved person, at both the personal as well as the institutional or ritual level.

Although anticipatory grieving may be regarded as the first psychological task to face the mother of an ill newborn, it may be that this process begins even earlier. I have been with mothers beginning to grieve before their baby is even born, when they show signs of going into labour at twenty-four or twenty-six weeks' gestation. The negative potential of anticipatory grieving emerges when the emotional reactions to the birth of an at-risk newborn, such as depression and mourning, may jeopardise the mother's relationship with her healthy new baby (Richards, 1983; Vera, 2003).

Anticipatory grieving in the parents of ill newborns was established by Benfield and colleagues (1976) in their study of 101 couples whose babies had been admitted to a NICU. A questionnaire measuring the parents' level of grieving was completed by each of the parents when their child was discharged. Despite the effects of time on the parents' memories, almost all reacted in a way comparable with those parents whose baby had died. The questionnaire responses showed feelings and attitudes and reported behaviours which reflected all too clearly the confusion and ambivalence associated with hovering between developing affection and anticipatory grieving.

The vacillation within the mother as she tries to make sense of her fluctuating emotions can only be compounded by her reactions to the unpredictable changes in her baby's condition. The improvements and setbacks in her baby's progress may be compared with the roller-coaster effect which is a well-known feature of grieving.

Preparing the parents

While for some parents the birth of an ill baby and her admission to the NNU will be an earth-shattering catastrophe, for others it may be less unpredictable. The woman who has been regarded as 'high-risk' during her pregnancy and who, with her fetus, has been through intensive antenatal monitoring will have been prepared for a less than physiological outcome. She may have been admitted to the antenatal ward on a long-term basis, or she may have been undergoing monitoring in a day assessment unit. Either way, the opportunity was presented to prepare her for the likely care of her baby in the NNU. The NNU staff are able to meet with parents to discuss anxieties and potential problems and to arrange a visit to the area of the NNU where their baby is likely to be cared for (Greig, 1998, 2002). The neonatal nurse is ideally suited to introduce the parents to both the physical environment and some of the staff who will be caring for their baby. Adopting an appropriately cautious or encouraging approach, the nurse explains the techniques and equipment which may be used; she may even include the 'rogue's gallery', showing the unit's successes.

The benefits of preparing the parents for the admission of a baby to the NNU were investigated in a mixed-method study (Greig, 2002). This research project accessed sixty-four mothers and twenty-five fathers whose babies were newly admitted and applied the Spielberger State Trait Anxiety Inventory to assess their concerns about their situation. Additionally, a smaller number agreed to a semi-structured interview, which was analysed qualitatively. Focus group data were also collected from NNU nursing staff. Although the quantitative data did not show any benefits associated with 'being prepared', these parents did report that coping was easier. The researcher interpreted 'being prepared' widely, including personal and family experience of NNU care. The NNU nursing staff, however, interpreted the term more narrowly, referring only to the prenatal tour mentioned above.

Parental involvement in care

When caring for parents in the NNU we aim to provide a setting in which they are able to grieve their loss and form a close, loving relationship with their newborn. To help them to come to accept the reality of their situation, they may be gently encouraged to see, hold and care for their baby from her earliest moments. This involvement is thought to help them, if and when it becomes necessary, to grieve for a specific baby, rather than for some vague entity which they never knew and are unable to recall or visualise.

Kennell and Klaus (1982) were the first to show us the importance of emphasising to the mother the positive aspects of her involvement with baby care. Whereas she may feel incompetent or even fearful of harming her baby, we should explain the benefits of her contact with her baby. Thus, welcoming the involvement of the mother in her baby's care is essential. We have to ensure that caring interventions which she is able to perform, such as feeding, should be certain to be successful. Thus, we help her to build up her self-confidence and self-esteem, to ensure an emotional environment in which the mother–child relationship can flourish.

In comparison to the rhetoric articulated by Kennell and Klaus, Greig showed that the reality did not always match up. She found that the first contact had a tendency to be 'thwarted' (2002: 333) by, for example, the baby being in an incubator for transport. The opportunities for the mothers in this sample to 'meet' their babies in the NNU were subject to 'frustrating delays' due largely to organisational factors (2002: 335). Greig found that the parents' actual caring began hesitantly and gradually increased with encouragement from the staff. A major concern for the mothers was their physical and emotional need to hold their babies. Greig compares this need with the sensation of 'empty arms' reported by bereaved mothers.

Communication

Communication between staff and parents is crucial in this setting. We need to think about the information and support needs of the parents, their difficulty in accepting the 'bad news' and some practical aspects of facilitating communication. Redshaw and colleagues found that bereaved parents value being able to 'talk to' nursing staff (1996: 181). This may reflect the finding of these researchers' full sample, that 'senior nurses' and 'junior nurses' are found to be the most helpful staff in terms of offering explanations, advice, support and sympathy (1996: 169).

Information-giving

> The worst thing was not being told why she was in, what their diagnosis was, what happened in labour and whether she would be OK or not.
>
> (Redshaw *et al.*, 1996: 168)

The parents' need for information, as in this example, may challenge the staff's knowledge and communication skills.

A major study of decision-making at the beginning of life (McHaffie, 2001) was undertaken in the east of Scotland and shed new light on communication and information-giving in the NNU. The researcher aimed to investigate parents' and staff perceptions of the withdrawal and/or withholding of treatment for newborns. In-depth face-to-face interviews at three months and thirteen months after the baby's death drew on the parents' experiences and opinions. The study involved fifty-nine sets of bereaved parents (fifty-eight mothers and forty-nine fathers). In this study 'communication problems were by far the commonest cause of dissatisfaction' among parents (2001: 65) and related largely to the lack of information. Parents devised ingenious tactics to obtain information, which would be admirable were it not that these people were beginning to grieve the forthcoming loss of their baby. The 'long silences' (2001: 65), during which no information was forthcoming, may have been associated with organisational matters, but assumed the dimensions of an ordeal. Other communication problems related to the recipient being unsupported, the information or reassurance proving incorrect, the ambivalence of the information and the variety of information-givers.

Information-giving styles were criticised by McHaffie's informants on the grounds of, for example, the public nature of the delivery or the steady delivery of small parcels of disappointment when the parent earnestly sought the complete picture. A potentially helpful 'rule of thumb' to guide the highly individual matter of information-giving is that the informer should 'be honest but not cruel' (Richards and Hawthorne, 1999: 67). In terms of basic information provision, we should initially prepare the parents for the baby's appearance and the battery of equipment surrounding her.

Later, the parents need to be encouraged to share their concerns about their role and their baby's progress, while information-giving continues. The verbal information given to the parents at their baby's admission may be supplemented and reinforced by a booklet covering similar areas. This information will be further enhanced by subsequent verbal information, notices, information boards and leaflets produced by the NNU staff and by organisations such as SANDS (Redshaw *et al.*, 1996: 170). Being with the new family or being absent requires that we balance the need to be supportive with the intimacy of their developing relationship.

Breaking bad news

When we inform parents of the anticipated death of their newborn, we need to take account of our own feelings of disappointment and failure as well as the parents' grief. The difficulties which we encounter when breaking bad news are aggravated by the possibility that the staff who face this situation are unlikely to be the most highly experienced. The problems feature prominently and frequently in the literature. This prominence suggests, though, that the difficulties are far from being resolved, despite educational interventions to remedy them (Farrell *et al.*, 2001).

In her authoritative study, McHaffie (2001) examined carefully how the news of the baby's vulnerable state reached the parents. All too often this sad news was given either to one parent alone or to another relative. The news was usually given by one of the medical staff, the exceptions being an advanced nurse practitioner and a police officer. The parents who were alone when the news was given resented this, not just because they were unsupported, but because of their perception of a conspiracy against them.

McHaffie's respondents described the nature of the news they were given. A large proportion actually seem to have been satisfied to have been told 'unequivocally that there was nothing more that could be done' (2001: 61). For other parents the picture emerged more gradually on the basis of investigations, which seems to have allowed the parents to adjust to the worsening prognosis. Particularly difficult was the experience of parents whose impressions were based on rather vague discussions and uncertainties which continued for, in some cases, months. The most difficult situation was when parents were initially reassured about the diagnosis, only later to find that it was incorrect. The parents' perceptions of how well the information-giving had been handled varied considerably. While many of McHaffie's respondents were satisfied, a number said it had been handled badly. There was variation, also, between their perceptions of the different hospitals.

Difficulty with breaking bad news was researched among Canadian medical staff, and certain areas to address were suggested (Dosanjh *et al.*, 2001). First is the verbal delivery, which should include, along with empathy and summary, validating and clarifying to maximise understanding. Their second area is the non-verbal aspects, such as posture, eye contact and time management.

Their final area covers the recipients' need for support, for example family availability and identifying common ground.

Facilitating communication

Parents' anxieties relate to both the welfare of their baby and to their own functioning as parents. Self-doubt may inhibit parents from seeking information about or contact with their child, so it is essential that NNU staff should 'go the extra mile' in order to ensure that the parents do keep in touch. This may be by providing a free telephone line through which parents may obtain up-to-date information from NNU staff about progress (Benfield *et al.*, 1978). Similarly, personal family contact (McHaffie, 1992) may be encouraged by genuine twenty-four-hour visiting, without anxiety-escalating delays before being allowed to enter the NNU (Richards and Hawthorne, 1999).

Communication between parents

The feelings of isolation engendered in each of the parents of an ill newborn make it unsurprising that their relationship undergoes considerable strain. Their difficulty in sharing their feelings about their experience is compounded by this stress.

The parents' inability to communicate with each other about the death of their baby was identified by McHaffie (2001: 267). For many of her informants, the research interview at about three months after the death was the first time that the couple had shared their feelings. Thus, the presence of a third party may be beneficial.

The couples in McHaffie's study went through a series of stages in their relationships which were reflected in different forms of communication. The parents reported that shortly after the death of the baby they experienced an unusual closeness, which the researcher compares with a 'honeymoon' (2001: 268). For a majority of couples, this intensity in their relationship had disappeared by the time of the second interview.

With the ending of the honeymoon a semblance of 'normality' returned to their communication styles. An important aspect of their post-bereavement communication was each partner's tendency to hide their feelings from the other. This may have been done for their own benefit, perhaps to reduce their feelings of guilt, or for the other's, such as to protect a partner perceived as vulnerable. Each partner's different style of grieving was a source of aggravation to the other. This potential for disharmony related to the father's different approach to demonstrating his grief. His partner's misreading of his silence led her to believe that she was quite alone in her sorrow. These misunderstandings gave rise to dissonance which, not infrequently, threatened the couple's relationship. This threat to the continuation of the relationship was not ameliorated by the presence of living children in the family (2001: 271). As well as this unfortunate outcome, the couple may have found that their loss may have brought some positive effects, such as getting their values into a better perspective, including strengthening their relationship, reducing discord and facilitating more open communication.

McHaffie's observation of a threat to the couple's relationship is applied more widely by Singg (2003: 885), who argues that the quality of interparental communication before their bereavement determines their adjustment and the survival of their relationship. Unfortunately, the basis of this observation is not given.

The care of the dying baby and her family

The care of the grieving family in the NNU has changed to become more sensitive and may be continuing to so develop.

In the past carers have sought to 'over-protect' the bereaved mother, by hiding the extent of her baby's difficulties. Whether it is actually the mother who is being protected is questionable, as the carers may be protecting themselves by avoiding embarrassing displays of overt grief. This 'over-protection' may also appear in the mother being discouraged from attending the funeral and having her baby equipment put away for her.

Dissatisfaction with the traditional tendency to 'over-protect' the mother served to initiate the research project which 'opened up' this topic and eventually increased parental involvement in NNUs (Kennell *et al.*, 1970). Twenty mothers who had had physical contact with their live newborns agreed to be involved after the babies survived between one hour and twelve days. The interviews focused on the birth experience and the baby's death, followed (for thirteen mothers) by a questionnaire. A grief score was calculated for each mother and was correlated with her experience.

As well as showing that mothers encounter no ill-effects attributable to touching or holding their dying babies, this study indicated that hospital policies regarding these mothers' care needed attention. Contact with the mothers of healthy babies was unwelcome and, although the grieving mother could deal with other mothers' casual enquiries, the 'awkward moments' due to staff ignorance were seriously disturbing.

Optimism led the parents to interpret casual remarks from junior medical staff as predicting survival. This interpretation included some elements of magical thinking – 'If the baby survives for – days, he will not die.' The parents were frequently and tragically disappointed.

This study discounted earlier assumptions that mother-love suddenly develops when a mother sees or touches her newborn, by demonstrating affectional ties well in advance of seeing or having physical contact. Previous practices, such as using what has become known as the 'rugby pass approach' to hastily remove stillborn babies from their mothers' presence or discouraging mothers' access to their sick or dying babies, were shown to be unhelpful. By addressing its social dimensions, these researchers showed us that the death of a newborn is something other than simply a medical event.

The future – In the same way as the care of the mother of the stillborn baby has changed to become more sensitive, it would seem logical that the principles of palliative care should be applied in the care of the newborn who is dying. The possibility of such care being available, however, appears uncertain (Pierucci *et al.*, 2001). The principles of palliative care have been summarised in the following terms:

1 Affirms life and regards dying as a normal process
2 Neither hastens nor postpones death
3 Provides relief from pain and other distressing symptoms
4 Integrates the psychological and spiritual aspects of care
5 Offers a support system to help [the baby] live as actively as possible until death
6 Offers a support system to help [the family] cope . . . in their own bereavement

(O'Neill and Fallon, 1997: 801)

Although the latter part of the first principle is clearly not relevant to neonatal care, it may be suggested that the remaining principles are highly applicable. Pierucci and his colleagues undertook a retrospective review of the use of a neonatal palliative care service in one US paediatric centre (2001). In a four-year period, 196 babies were found to have died under the age of one year. The researchers found that only 13 per cent (n=25) of the bereaved families had been referred for consultation with the nurse-led palliative care service. There were no significant differences between the referred and the non-referred groups, as the diagnoses of the babies whose families used the palliative care service matched those of the other babies.

These researchers found that the advice offered by the palliative care staff fell into four categories:

1 **Optimal environment** for supporting neonatal death was found to be somewhere other than the NNU. Following a palliative care consultation the baby was likely to spend fewer days in the NNU and was less likely to die there. Some of the families referred for consultation took their baby home to die, although data are not available on this group.
2 **Advance directive** planning had implications for end-of-life decision-making (see page 123). The babies whose family was referred for palliative care consultation were less likely to be subjected to cardio-pulmonary resuscitation (CPR) and significantly less likely to be administered cardiac stimulant medication and mechanical ventilation.
3 **Comfort and medical care** in babies following palliative care consultations featured, not just the administration of narcotic drugs, but also a reduction in invasive investigations and interventions. These included taking blood specimens, endotracheal intubation and nasogastric feeding. The presence or absence of not to be resuscitated (NTBR) orders

did not affect the support offered to the families in making funeral arrangements.

4 **Psychosocial support** was more prominent in the families of babies who had been referred. This does not mean that that support was greater or more effective, but it was better organised and documented. These researchers also found that consultations with faith leaders and social workers were significantly more frequent.

These findings resonate with the earlier work of Harmon and colleagues (1984) who implemented palliative care in a NICU, which resulted in, first, aggressive medical interventions being used more cautiously, second, more attention being given to a comfortable atmosphere in the unit and, third, a greater focus on the needs of the family, such as a family room for being with a dying or dead baby.

Social and staff support

The social dimensions of the care of newborns extend far beyond the nuclear family and the staff. This was demonstrated in a study of social support for the parents of babies in a NICU (McHaffie, 1992) which focused on the role of grandparents. Four main components of social support are usually differentiated: emotional support, esteem-building, instrumental support and information-giving. Using questionnaires, McHaffie sought the views of parents and grandparents, as well as NNU staff. In this study she highlighted some of the 'mismatches' between staff expectations and grandparents' actual support. Their role is greatly and widely undervalued by staff, particularly by our medical colleagues. If we are to provide a milieu in which parents can relate to their newborn, it is essential to encourage and utilise their informal support system.

Although I look at staff support in the context of loss generally in Chapter 10, I mention it briefly here because of specific relevant research and because of the implications of the unique NNU environment. The problems for NNU staff when a baby dies relate to not only their professional feelings of failure, but also the grief for the death of a person with whom, over a period of hours, days or weeks, they have developed a caring relationship.

Coping mechanisms

A 'chronic' baby died who'd been on the unit for over five months. I went to the funeral. Since then no one has asked how I feel and no one has offered any support whatsoever. It has been left to non-nursing friends to pick me up and encourage me to stick at neonatal nursing.
(Informant, in Redshaw *et al.*, 1996: 182)

On the basis of such data, Redshaw recommends that a 'more structured' form of staff support is needed in the NNU. One form of support would be staff support groups, whose problems and benefits Richards and Hawthorne (1999) mention in the context of some of the challenges faced by NNU staff. These challenges include coping with the psychological stress, pain and conflict engendered through caring for newborns. Denial and avoidance feature prominently among the short-term coping mechanisms, which have caused problems in the establishment of support groups. Magical thinking and intuition may also feature, such as the 'unlucky incubator'. Staff also use projection and splitting, involving blaming others (including objects) for events for which they feel responsible. Examples include blaming the obstetrician, the ward staff or the 'other' hospital for less than optimal care.

Less experienced and junior staff identify with the parents in their feelings of inadequacy, incompetence and ignorance. Likewise, feelings of distress in the staff may be uncomfortably similar to those that they imagine are being felt by the baby. Feelings of rivalry, perhaps to be expected in a new mother faced by super-competent staff, are also experienced by those staff. This reflects attachment which is an inevitable consequence of the long-term close contact of staff with ill newborns, which may be aggravated as primary nursing becomes more widespread.

Decision-making: initiating and discontinuing treatment

In providing care for the family and their newborn we aim to sustain life and alleviate suffering. Ordinarily these aims are mutually compatible, but sometimes there may be conflict. An example is the low birth weight baby whose healthy development is jeopardised by the various insults to which she is vulnerable. Questions arise about whether and for how long treatment should be continued, about who should make the decision and how it should be made. In some countries these decisions have been assumed by the legislature, but in the UK the situation is less clear. Although euthanasia may be relevant, I am focusing on treatment-related decisions because, although the outcome may be similar, the decisions, intentionality and procedures are not.

Initiation of treatment

The seriously ill newborn in the NNU may have been resuscitated in the birthing room or she may have begun breathing spontaneously. Either way, her independent existence has become established. Any other course of action would be inappropriate, because the labour ward is not the ideal place to make unexpected life-and-death decisions, due to the limited time to either confer with the parents or make a complete assessment of the baby's condition. Unfortunately, when the baby is transferred to the NNU a sequence of interventions has begun which assumes a momentum of its own. In their study of aggressive neonatal care, Guillemin and Holmstrom

(1986) describe this form of incrementalism as the 'all or none' law. It is necessary to question whether this policy constitutes care of any kind or, even less, humane care.

Resource implications

Bound up with initiation/continuation of treatment are issues relating to resource allocation. Without disregarding the financial costs of caring for a sick newborn for possibly a matter of months, I should also consider what other 'opportunities' may be foregone. By providing NNU care for a baby born at twenty-four weeks, we may be denying care to three babies born at thirty-two weeks. The question needs to be raised of whether decision-making on a 'first come, first served' basis is ideal.

End of life decision-making

It is possible that who makes the decision about continuing or limiting treatment may affect the outcome of that decision. Medical staff focus on the immediate situation and the problems as they present in the NNU, whereas their nursing colleagues are better able to adopt a 'holistic view' (Guillemin and Holmstrom, 1986). Thus, nurses think of the baby becoming a child and a person in a social context and the family resources required to care for someone growing up with potentially severe disabilities. This point is not unrelated to the earlier 'incrementalist' argument, because staff who have worked hard to sustain a newborn may have difficulty in abandoning all the effort and emotion that they have invested in her.

The involvement of parents in treatment decision-making has been criticised on the grounds that such responsibility is hard to bear (McHaffie *et al.*, 2001). Whether parents do share this responsibility or whether medical practitioners behave in a benevolently paternalistic way featured in the research project by McHaffie and her colleagues (2001). This paternalism materialises to some extent in McHaffie's finding that 'only 3% of doctors and 6% of nurses' thought that parents should be given the responsibility for the 'ultimate decision' (2001: 396). In spite of this, a large proportion (n=45: 42 per cent) of the parents of babies whose treatment had been withdrawn felt that they had actually made the decision.

In terms of the ensuing feelings, the parents in McHaffie's study were generally satisfied with their involvement in making the decision. Benfield *et al.*, on the other hand, compared the grieving of nineteen parents who had contributed to the treatment limitation decision with the grieving of twenty-one parents whose babies had received total care (1978). The mothers of the limited treatment babies demonstrated significantly less anger, irritability and 'wanting to be left alone'. The fathers in the limited treatment group encountered less sleeplessness, irritability, depression, crying and loss of appetite. Thus, while some parents may avoid such involvement, well-informed parents are able to contribute to taxing decisions about treatment and go on to adjust healthily to their loss.

Although these ensuing feelings appear to be satisfactory for a large proportion of parents, the question remains of whether a more suitable framework might be operationalised for the more difficult decisions. It might be necessary to contemplate the introduction of different structures, such as an ethics committee. A consensus in which the rights, needs, responsibilities and feelings of all concerned are taken into account would appear to be ideal. Transparency in this form of decision-making would maintain the confidence of all who are involved and, particularly important, the public.

Care after the decision to discontinue treatment

In the study by McHaffie (2001) the parents were variably prepared for what would happen after treatment was discontinued. The duration of the baby's dying was most frequently predicted as being 'quick'. Perhaps because of this expectation, the parents were often shocked at how long the baby actually took to die. In view of this disconcertingly long time period it is unsurprising that different reactions were encountered in the parents. Some of the parents had been assured, prior to treatment being discontinued, that the baby would not suffer. Even more (n=15 couples: 25 per cent) had been told that narcotic analgesic drugs would be used in sufficient doses to ensure that this was so. Some parents understood the respiratory depressant effects of these medications. A couple whose baby took thirty-six hours to die reflected: 'But even if you knew it was going to be thirty-six hours, what could you do apart from giving a whacking great dose of morphine immediately she came off the ventilator?' (2001: 157). Another reaction among the parents during the babies' period of dying was to consider reversing the treatment limitation decision. This prospect is not unreasonable when the parents realised that the baby had a much firmer hold on life than they had been led to believe: 'I felt because he was putting up such a strong fight, there was a couple of times I contemplated reversing [the decision and putting the tube back in]. It was really distressing. It felt like a lifetime' (2001: 156).

The parents continue to be involved whenever possible in a private setting, together with other chosen family members. Supporting the parents through the baby's dying and laying-out is essential, in the hope that they appreciate the naturalness of death and its fundamental importance to life.

The setting in which care happens

Up to this point in this chapter we have been thinking about the processes and events which take place in the NNU. These include beginning relationships, ending others, loving, supporting as well as making difficult decisions. I would like now to focus on the environment in which all these events happen and which inevitably affects them, starting with the intimate environment in which the baby is treated and moving on to the more general environment in which parents and staff interact.

Touch and handling

The benefits of tactile stimulation to a newborn are well established; likewise, parental care involves handling as part of affectionate social interaction. Emphasising the importance of rest for LBW and sick newborns, Wolke (1987a) reminds us of the iatrogenic effects of excessive manipulation during monitoring and other procedures, including hypoxaemia, bradycardia, apnoea and behavioural distress. In their intensive observational study of eleven extremely LBW babies, Werner and Conway (1990) recorded contacts during twenty hours of care. Disconcertingly, these researchers found that the most vulnerable babies were exposed to the greatest number of disturbing contacts, to the extent that those with a 'Minimal Touch' instruction were disturbed approximately twice as often as those without. These researchers challenge neonatal nurses to plan and coordinate their care in order to minimise disruption and maximise comfort activities.

The purely physical benefits of the LBW newborn's immediate environment are considered by Turrill (1992). She discusses the effects of being born prematurely on the infant's perception of and relationship with her immediate environment. This baby is deprived of pressure from the uterine walls which the fetus ordinarily experiences due, first, to the walls' increasing contractility and, second, to the relative reduction in amniotic fluid. The effect of extra-uterine gravity has more marked effects on the relatively hypotonic newborn musculature. Thus, normal sensorimotor development is impeded, unless deliberate precautions are taken to imitate the natural phenomena by correct positioning and other interventions.

A way of controlling the neonatal environment which has attracted considerable media and some research attention since it was first introduced in Colombia in 1978 is kangaroo mother care (KMC) (Conde-Agudelo *et al.*, 2004). By effectively 'marsupialising' the low birth weight newborn between the mother's breasts, this intervention is intended to reduce the need for costly and potentially iatrogenic neonatal care. The newborn maintains skin-to-skin contact and frequent and exclusive breastfeeding. While the systematic review by Conde-Agudelo and colleagues suggests that newborn morbidity may be reduced by KMC, the quality of the research to date is not high enough to be able to advocate this form of care. Similarly, KMC's close relative, skin-to-skin contact, has been credited with a number of more or less tangible benefits. Skin-to-skin, though, has been shown to be beneficial in increasing the likelihood of breastfeeding being successfully established and reducing neonatal crying. There appear to be no significant short-term or long-term disadvantages to this intervention. Again, though, the quality of the research methods prevents any more concrete conclusions (Anderson *et al.*, 2004).

A form of care which is certainly conceptually appealing derives from the work of Heidi Als (Richards and Hawthorne, 1999). Als argues that care which is developmentally appropriate should be provided for low birth weight babies. This 'developmental care' provides the newborn with an environment similar to that which it would be enjoying, had the birth not intervened. While Als's NIDCAP (Neonatal Individualised Developmental Care and Assessment Program) has been subjected to considerable research attention, Symington and Pinelli (2004) consider the case for developmental care to be 'unproven' in view of the plethora of interventions involved. A diametrically opposed view is presented by Ruiz (2001), who argues that neonatal nurses who do not practise developmental care are practising to a less than ethical standard. In view of this huge divergence of views and the potential for limited health care resources to be misappropriated, a serious evaluation of implementing this form of care may be overdue.

The wider environment

Although they avoid the words, Werner and Conway (1990) demonstrated the negative stressors which are inadvertently applied by carers in the NNU. These cause physical stress as well as psychological stress through interrupting sleep and rest. Richards and Hawthorne (1999) outline the implications of certain aspects of care in the NNU, including the well-known effects of continuous noise and bright light (Wolke, 1987a, 1987b). These authors argue persuasively the disadvantages for the baby of a 'task oriented' organisation of care. Although the more individualised approaches to care may be less attractive in organisational terms, they carry benefits for the individual baby and staff member.

Changing attitudes

Concerns about the harmful effects of NNUs on newborn development underlie research by Becker *et al.* (1991). They discuss the stressful NNU environment and its potential for impeding learning. These researchers also advocate an individualised developmental approach to care. To evaluate this approach they designed an experimental study comparing growth and behavioural organisation outcome measures in two groups of very LBW babies. The first group of twenty-one newborns acted as controls. The second, experimental group of twenty-four were cared for by nurses who had been educated both didactically and individually to reduce environmental stressors by:

- limiting light and sound
- providing comfort during interventions, such as by using a dummy (soother or pacifier)
- promoting sleep/wake organisation by planning/clustering interventions

- giving postural support through the use of 'nesters'
- encouraging non-nutritive sucking while tube-feeding.

Newborns in the experimental group encountered fewer respiratory and feeding problems, lower morbidity, shorter admission times and better behavioural organisation. These outcomes indicate that education of nurses to take account of environmental and psychological factors does affect newborn well-being.

The NNU environment

Considerable research has focused on the setting in which care of the LBW and ill newborn is provided. The hazards which have been identified and the outcomes which have been measured relate to the well-being of the newborn. The NNU as a working environment has been given less attention. While the emotional environment has been addressed earlier in this chapter (see 'Social and staff support'), the physical environment is the focus here. In the course of a study of neonatal care, Redshaw and colleagues (1996) considered the health and sickness absence of neonatal nursing staff. Using indicators such as body mass index, smoking and alcohol consumption, these researchers found that neonatal nurses compare not unfavourably with similar groups and with the general population of women.

The physical environment was assessed using a checklist during the researchers' visits to the NNUs. This assessment showed that, whereas the entrance is more likely to be gloomy (n=10: 42 per cent), rather than bright or neutral, the NNU itself tends to be bright (n=15: 63 per cent). The less than welcoming nature of the entrance is reinforced by the usual need to ring a bell and wait to be allowed to enter (n=17: 71 per cent). Whereas most of the units visited were well furnished in terms of curtains/blinds and suitable accommodation for parents, only a minority were wallpapered (n=11: 46 per cent).

Redshaw and her colleagues found that more of the nursing staff were dissatisfied with the physical environment than the parents. For example while 51.5 per cent of nursing staff considered that the lighting needed improvement, only 8.6 per cent of parents thought so. Similarly, the noise level was criticised by 49.4 per cent of nurses, but only 13.1 per cent of parents. Considerably more agreement was found on the subject of space, with 53.8 per cent of parents thinking it could be improved compared with 68.7 per cent of nurses. As one parent stated: 'The rooms were so cramped there was hardly any space to put the screen for feeding, and no room for visitors' (Redshaw et al., 1996: 174).

Summary

'All human life is there' in the NNU and, one might add, a lot more besides.

I have shown that the NNU is for living, loving and dying, for finding and losing, for helping to live as well as allowing to die. These activities continue to happen regardless of the environment. I have shown the efforts which are being made to improve the environment for the babies beginning their lives there and what is being done to improve the experience of their parents and family. Whether we have the healthiest environment in which the staff are able to facilitate all these activities is less certain.

9   The death of a mother

The death of a mother, or maternal mortality, is a topic which, despite its relative rarity in developed countries, brings with it a multiplicity of issues. It is not possible to do justice to these issues in just one chapter. For this reason, I attempt to introduce the topic and demonstrate its significance, with a particular emphasis on the care providers. Because maternal death raises very different issues in developing countries, the focus here is primarily on those which are relatively affluent.

The introduction to this topic touches on some of these issues by addressing historical phenomena and their representation in artistic form. I then give brief attention to the international situation to indicate the global significance of these concerns. The experience of the family is briefly considered next, followed by the issues raised for midwifery staff. There is some discussion of one approach to resolve the problem of maternal mortality. The conclusion shows that there are certain areas urgently in need of research.

Because maternal death is appropriately regarded as a serious challenge for health care systems, policy makers and health care provision, it is ordinarily viewed in terms of being a public health problem. This is quite proper in areas where maternal death carries momentous implications for the population as a whole. In more developed countries, though, the death of a mother is likely to be investigated on an individual basis to identify any avoidable factors from which health care providers may learn and, hopefully, improve practice (Lewis and Drife, 2004: 4). In these situations it is possible and may be helpful to take a more personal approach to the issues raised by the death of a mother. For this reason, throughout this chapter, I endeavour to adopt a less objective and a more human approach to this topic than ordinarily features in the literature. An example is Loudon's beginning to his admirable book on maternal death, which comprises the story of such a tragedy and serves to remind the reader of what lies 'behind the analysis of numbers, trends, causes, and factors' (1992: 3). It is unfortunate, though, that his subsequent text addresses only the analysis.

The historical context

The dangerousness of childbearing, especially in historical times, invariably features prominently. An example is found in the influential work of Stone (1977) on the English family between 1500 and 1800. He blames the 'very dangerous experience' (1977: 79) which was childbirth on the low standard of midwifery care. In support of this accusation he cites the high level of mortality among the 'squirarchy', perhaps not realising that such relatively wealthy women would be more likely to be attended by physicians than by midwives. In spite of this inappropriate blame, the perception of the dangerousness of childbearing still stands. Whether this perception is justified historically is difficult to confirm because, as Loudon (1992: 19) demonstrates, the calculation of historical maternal mortality is far from being a precise science. Schofield (1986) takes Loudon's argument a stage further by denying that English maternal mortality rates were at such an unacceptably high level: 'The risk of dying in childbed was no greater than the risk she ran every year of dying from infectious disease and a whole variety of other causes' (1986: 260). Unfortunately, Schofield's argument relies heavily on Swedish data, without explaining its relevance to the English context.

Despite this, Houlbrooke, in his work on the English family in the fifteenth to seventeenth centuries, estimates that the overall maternal mortality rate was 'twenty-five per thousand birth events' (1984: 129). The variability in these rates, though, becomes apparent in the work of Marshall (2004) who found that the rate for two parishes in the city of Edinburgh from 1739 to 1769 was almost twice as high as the rate in the City of London (3.7 per cent and 2 per cent of all female deaths respectively).

Further support to the historical dangerousness of childbearing may be found in the epitaphs which were carved on the women's gravestones. One example recorded by Monteith is found on a monument in Greyfriars Churchyard in Edinburgh:

> To the memory of his dearest wife Elizabeth Gillespie, daughter to the most learned Mr George Gillespie, minister at Edinburgh, and who was learned far above her sex: and having brought forth no daughter, died in the birth of the seventh son, 5 March 1681 and of her age the 33 year.
>
> (1704: 13–14).

As well as epitaphs on gravestones, the more educated members of society were able to write of their sorrow at the death of a mother. This is demonstrated in a letter written on 2 August 1733 by John Campbell to his father Patrick Campbell of Barcaldine. The letter announced the death of their sister/daughter respectively: 'yesternight about nine of the clock after being delivered of a dead child'. John Campbell concluded that they must console themselves by thinking of: 'the character and the pretty familie of childeren she hes left. The funeral will be next Tuesday. Her husband, poor Ardchattan, is inconsolable and begs to have everything done in the genteelest manner (Campbell, 1733). While this woman, whose name is uncertain, clearly had had other living children, first-time mothers were no less vulnerable. John Clerk of Penicuik, near Edinburgh, wrote of his experience of the death of his wife, Lady Margaret Stewart, in December 1701 after a lengthy and harrowing labour and the birth of a boy. They had only been married on 6 March that year. All the most prominent physicians had been summoned from Edinburgh to attend her:

> They took all the pains about her they cou'd think of, but I am afraied they were too hasty in their operations, by which she lost a vast deal of blood. The placenta, it seems was adhering to the uterus and this they thought themselves oblidged to bring away by force. Her cries were so piercing to me in the next room that it wou'd be very difficult for anybody to conceive the vast agony they put me in.
>
> (Gray, 1892: 39–42)

These 'frequent tragedies' (Marshall, 1983: 114) were familiar and raised anxieties for all involved, to the extent that childbirth in the seventeenth century has been compared with an 'excruciatingly painful dress rehearsal for death' (Houlbrooke, 1998: 68). While a pilgrimage to a nearby shrine (Marshall, 1983: 42) may have allayed some anxiety, this state of mind may not have been ideal for embarking on labour.

Representations of the death of a mother

Although some regard them as a modern phenomenon, pictorial representations of babies who have not survived have long been used as a source of comfort to a grieving family (Mander and Marshall, 2003). Pictorial records of mothers who have died, though, are considerably less common. The reasons for their rarity may only be surmised. While, as has been shown, neither event was unusual in numerical terms, it may be that concern for the child was greater because the welfare of her/his eternal soul was less assured than that of the mother's.

The seventeenth century monument to Lady Jane Crewe (d. 1639) is displayed in Westminster Abbey, London (see Figure 9.1). The sculptor of this wall monument made unique use of a panel carved in relief to show a family near the deathbed of a newly delivered mother. In the background is the woman on her deathbed, while in the foreground the bereaved family focuses its attention on ensuring the survival of the apparently living newborn baby. The father seated to the right is not involved with the baby care, as he appears to be having difficulty coming to terms with his loss and wondering how he will manage to raise his growing family single-handedly (Houlbrooke, 1998: 349).

A particularly perplexing painting is *The Saltonstall Family* (1636–7) by

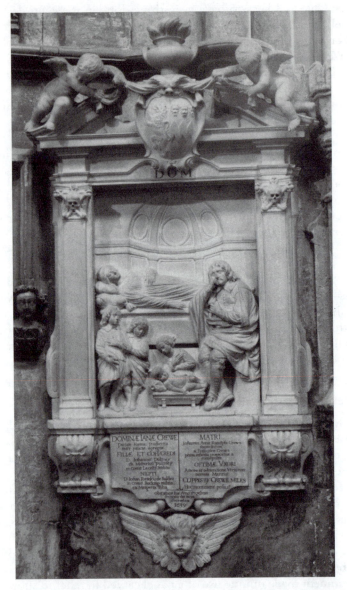

Figure 9.1 The monument to Lady Jane Crewe in Westminster Abbey, London (Copyright: Dean and Chapter of Westminster Abbey. Reproduced with kind permission)

David des Granges (1611/13–?1675). Hand in hand with the paterfamilias, Sir Richard Saltonstall, stand two small children. In the background, on her deathbed, lies his first wife, pointing towards the toddlers. Seated at the bedside, though, is another young woman holding a swaddled baby. Hearn

(2001) suggests that the young woman is Saltonstall's second wife with one of their children. While sometimes taken to represent family unity and continuity, this decidedly unsettling painting may have other more sinister meanings.

The painting by Edvard Munch (1863–1944) entitled *The Dead Mother* (1899–1900) is less familiar than his *The Scream/The Cry*, but is only marginally less disturbing. It shows a small child, who probably represents the painter as a child, with his mother's dead body in the background. Although the child in this painting is clearly not a newborn baby, its raw emotion, characteristic of Munch's work, captures the overwhelming sense of loss when a mother dies.

The international situation

In developed countries, the maternal mortality rate fell during and after the Second World War to reach what may be regarded as an irreducible minimum in the final decades of the twentieth century. That the figure is no longer falling may be associated with the following factors. First, due to health and social care advances women with serious health problems, such as cancer, are able and likely to become pregnant. This may be associated with untimely death (Larkin, 1990). The widespread trend of women to delay childbearing means that certain conditions of maturity or even old age, such as certain cancers, are likely to feature more frequently and may cause death (Keleher *et al.*, 2002).

World Health Organisation figures (2004) show that the maternal mortality ratio (the number of maternal deaths per 100,000 live births) in developed countries fell from twenty-one to twenty between the years 1995 and 2000. This may support the suggestion mentioned above that an irreducible minimum may have been reached. The overall ratio for developing regions, though, remained static during this period at 440. This static figure serves to conceal, though, the increasing ratio in south-central Asia from 410 to 520. Thus, it is apparent that, while maternal mortality may be being addressed in some areas, there are others where the numbers are not only disconcertingly great, but are also increasing.

Using the situation in Afghanistan as an example, del Valle (2004) argues that a broad-brush approach is necessary if the problem of maternal mortality is to be resolved. This includes addressing matters of gender politics, women's rights and women's education. He considers that a comprehensive and sustainable public health plan is needed. This must include the establishment of an infrastructure which supports the provision of services in not only urban centres but also isolated rural communities. He goes on to argue that the public health reforms which were introduced to industrialised countries in the nineteenth century, such as safe water, adequate shelter and effective sanitation/sewerage, have still to be achieved in many developing areas.

The experience of the family

It should come as no surprise that the effects of the death of the mother on the family are not well addressed. It has been shown that even health care providers are unable to accept the reality of maternal death (Mander, 2001a), so how much more difficult must this concept be for those without their experience? Research has, probably appropriately, sought to remedy the causes of maternal death, rather than resolve the problems raised for those indirectly affected. In this section the assumption is being made that the woman who died was in a heterosexual relationship.

One research project which does serve to inform the family implications was undertaken as part of a programme addressing issues relating to maternal mortality in Mexico (Reyes Frausto *et al.*, 1998). This is a country which, in spite of a hospital birth rate of over 90 per cent and well-developed obstetric services, has a maternal mortality ratio of 114 per 100,000 in Mexico City (Koblinsky and Campbell, 1999). The research by Reyes Frausto and her colleagues involved interviews with members of the dead woman's family. In those families in which the baby survived, a second interview was undertaken when the baby was one year old. The data were analysed quantitatively. These researchers were successful in identifying the extent of the family breakdown or 'disintegration' (1998: 433) following the woman's death. They also showed the way in which the children in the family were required to adopt new roles and any financial difficulties were exacerbated. These latter changes were most marked in families where the mother had been poorly or unsupported. These Mexican researchers found that those babies who survived became integrated into the family of their grandparents. This is a reflection, first, of the older siblings' limited ability to manage the new roles which they had been required to adopt. Second, it reflects the father's difficulty in overcoming his loss in order to meet the needs of his young family.

The problems which the grandparents and other family members may encounter in situations where the mother is lost and the father absent have been documented in historical terms (Marshall, 1976). In 1707 the grandmother of the baby Thomas, Lord Erskine, wrote to other family members that she was 'mightily perplexed' (1976: 13) about the baby's feeding problems. Finding and retaining a suitable wet nurse was a major headache. The medical advisor, a Dr Pitcairn, was a mixed blessing as his ideas about feeding were definite and different from the grandmother's, but he was able to locate a suitable wet nurse.

The grandparents' assumption of responsibility for the care of the baby is not just an historical phenomenon. In her case-study of the effects of maternal death on the family, Cooke (1990) describes the grandparental role in terms similar to those applying to the eighteenth-century Scottish nobility; her main focus, however, is on the partner's loss. The study by Ferri (1975) found that only one-quarter of bereaved fathers located a parent substitute.

It was found to be the father's age that determined whether this should be a grandparent or another, with younger fathers relying on their parents. The question of who provides care for the child is likely to be a vexed one. Cooke outlines the difficulties in these arrangements including, first, the substitute carer adopting that role following a (possibly unwelcome) deathbed request. Second, the grandparents, while grieving their untimely loss, may find themselves taking on a role which they had been glad to relinquish many years earlier. Third, the father may resent the person who usurps the role of his partner in caring for their children.

In reviewing what it is that is lost, Cooke emphasises the secondary losses, such as loss of one part of the family income. She also raises the partner's 'loss of self', through the 'husband becoming a widower' (1990: 4) and the dissolution of the partnership. It is possible that the challenges of being 'forced' into lone fatherhood are greater than those faced by a father who chooses to maintain his parental responsibilities after the breakdown of a relationship.

In her chronological analysis of the child's reaction to the death of the mother, Cooke relies heavily on the research by Raphael (1982). This research project addressed the care of children who had known the parent who died. This is clear from the fact that the children were interviewed within 'the first few weeks' (1982: 133) of the death and none were under two years of age. It may be assumed that the children had formed a relationship with the parent who died and that such children would need to grieve and mourn the loss of their parent, albeit in a style which may differ from that manifested by adults. Because the relationship of a fetus/neonate is at best different, whether Raphael's account of grief behaviour applies to the child whose mother dies before, at the moment of or shortly after her birth is difficult to determine. Thus, while not underestimating the perceptiveness of small children to the emotional atmosphere surrounding them, it is necessary to conclude that the relevance of Raphael's study to maternal death is questionable.

The experience of the midwife

In her insightful paper, Cooke (1990) briefly introduces some of the issues for the midwife when a mother in her care dies. She mentions the confusion, the inappropriateness and the personal sense of failure and loss. Partly because of the need for more attention to this topic raised by Cooke's work, I undertook a research project which focused on the experience of the midwife when a woman in her care dies. The specifically support-related issues which emerged out of this study have been addressed in Chapter 10. In this section I describe the research project, before addressing the more general issues which arose.

A research project

The *research questions* were based on my limited personal experience, a review of the literature and the impressions gained through informal conversations (Mander, 2001b, 2004b). The first probed a previously unaddressed area: 'How does the experience of caring for a mother who dies affect the midwife?' The second question sought to provide more appropriate help to the midwife with this experience: 'What interventions does the midwife identify as either helpful or unhelpful to her after she has cared for a mother who has died?' The third question aimed to find out whether midwives who had not had this experience shared the same ideas, whether the death of a mother was viewed differently and whether and how the potential for maternal death affected the midwife: 'Does the remote possibility of maternal death influence the practice of a midwife caring for a mother who is experiencing an uncomplicated pregnancy, childbirth or puerperium? If so in what way does this influence operate?'

A *qualitative approach* was clearly the only way to address such a sensitive and unmentionable topic. Phenomenology was chosen to access the experience of the midwife providing care. This approach permits a comprehensive account of the phenomenon to be created by viewing the lived experience through the other person's eyes (Stephenson and Corben, 1997). The phenomenological researcher seeks to suspend her personal beliefs and biases through 'bracketing' in order to accept more completely the experience which the informant recounts. The data analysis typically features a 'clustering' to develop themes which describe the phenomenon.

In order to *recruit* midwife informants, advertising would have been appropriate, but was prevented by lack of funds. The editor of a wide-circulation midwifery journal, however, was prepared to accept an item on this topic (Mander, 1999b). This item outlined the problem and the research and sought responses from suitably experienced midwives. Three methods of initial contact were suggested and details provided; these were telephone, post and email.

To *collect data*, telephone interviews were chosen due to lack of funding to travel to face-to-face interviews. Permission to tape-record was generally forthcoming, and was followed by transcription for analysis.

The interviews were semi-structured and, after the introductory sequence, the informant was asked to recount her experience. On the basis of this account and a rolling 'agenda' of questions, each midwife's experience was examined.

The interviews with the 'experienced' midwives, who had attended a mother who died, happened in the 'First Round'. A check on the full findings was planned to happen in the 'Second Round'. This comprised returning to re-interview some of the 'experienced' midwife informants to check on the data. In this round, midwives who had no experience of the death of a mother were also interviewed. Data were also collected through letters and by email messages.

A form of 'snowball sampling' (Morse, 1989) was used to recruit midwives who have not cared for a mother who has died. This ensured that these 'non-experienced' midwives were comparable, at least through geographical proximity, to those who were 'experienced'.

The *analysis of the data* was undertaken concurrently with the data collection/fieldwork. Each interview was compared with the previous ones and other existing data. The emerging themes were probed in subsequent interviews until it became apparent that no new aspect of a particular theme was being raised by the informants. This ongoing analysis of the data was supplemented by a further check of the transcripts after the completion of the fieldwork. This ensured that no nuances were overlooked.

Thirty-six midwife informants provided data. Of these thirty-two had experience of being associated with the care of a woman who had died. The Second Round comprised repeat interviews with three of the 'experienced' midwives who had been interviewed in the First Round. There were also interviews with four midwives who had no experience of caring for a mother who had died. Whereas the initial contact was by one of three methods, subsequent contacts were invariably by telephone.

I avoided collecting data about each midwife's personal background; this is because the focus of the study was on the midwife's perception of this experience and any effects which it may have on her and/or on her practice. In the same way, data were not specifically collected relating to the circumstances of the woman's death. Only those details necessary to understand the midwife's reaction were sought.

This study is limited in that it was an exploratory study. It aimed, primarily, to examine the meaning to the midwife of the experience of caring for a woman who died. While the qualitative research design is appropriate for an area about which little is written, there are limitations, such as the nature of the sample, which comprised volunteers. Thus, the findings are not generalisable.

A number of *ethical problems* were raised by this study. The first related to the absence of research ethics committee (REC) approval. I decided that such approval was unnecessary because the sample was a volunteer sample of healthy individuals. That the informants did not receive an information sheet or complete a consent form may be construed as infringements of their ethical rights. In spite, or perhaps because, of these omissions, the researcher endeavoured throughout each interview to empathise with the informant's reactions and to tailor the interview to limit any discomfort to her.

The first major theme which emerged was the *midwife's attitude* to the death of a mother. This manifested itself, first, in the 'experienced' midwives' inability to share their experience with those who were 'inexperienced':

The feelings were too raw to share. The affected group kept close together.

(Midwife 04)

The development of this 'in group', however, meant that those without this experience were treated as outsiders. This clearly prevents the 'inexperienced' midwife from learning from her 'experienced' colleagues. This exclusion may serve to aggravate the 'conspiracy of silence' which surrounds maternal death:

> Part of the problem is that people say it does not happen in this country. You don't think about it happening.
>
> (Midwife 08)

This concern was articulated very clearly by another midwife who was clearly uneasy about this silence and the element of superstitious or magical thinking associated with it:

> It's almost as if the subject doesn't exist. What's written is about a husband who's bereaved ... but there's nothing for maternal death. There just isn't enough mentioned about it. It's like a dark subject which we won't talk about in case it happens.
>
> RM: Do you think that's the reason for avoiding it?
>
> I think so. It's almost as if it jinxes you if you talk about it. Plus I don't think that people really know how to talk about maternal death. Even if it happens in a hospital, a sort of gloom and a pall sort of descends over the place, but nobody will kind of speak to the people involved. So as a result you're kind of left out there in the cold – no one talks to you about it at all. It's very strange actually.
>
> (Midwife 13)

It may be that these attitudes are not the healthiest way for the midwife to address this much-feared phenomenon. It is to be hoped that, in the same way as more open discussion has improved the care of the bereaved mother, more openness may be helpful to the midwife.

It is not impossible that these less than healthy attitudes may be being aggravated by another factor which was identified. This factor comprises the paradox between expectations of childbearing and the reality which the experienced midwives had encountered. Some of the midwives presented others' views of childbearing as naïve:

> Because the attitude is that it's pregnancy and that's OK and people don't die when they're young or of pregnancy.
>
> (Midwife 14)

I have found that students have actually asked me isn't midwifery a wonderful thing. And I say not always – when things go wrong it's not very nice at all. And that takes people by surprise.

(Midwife 19)

The direct entry students found the whole thing difficult because they thought they'd come into an area that was happy and it was turning out to be different from what they'd expected.

(Midwife 14)

What these lay people and students were encountering, though, was an experience which verged on a disaster in terms of its intensity, if not its extent. In the same way, the midwives found themselves unready to cope with the reality facing them:

No one had spoken to me at all about the situations leading to maternal death during my training. I think it was only mentioned occasionally and I was not at all prepared.

(Midwife 19)

Those midwives who did accept maternal death as a reality assumed that it happened to others:

So there's an enormous, a huge, sense of disbelief that it's happening and also because we are dealing with young fit women and y'know I do have the greatest respect for obstetricians. There's also a sense of the fact that Dr A or Dr B is there and really the woman will be all right. There aren't terribly many things that aren't solvable.

(Midwife 24)

I am sure you can appreciate that after ten years' practice I never expected to be involved with the death of a mother. I presumed that, as we were in the 1980s and I was working in a small maternity, that it just could not happen. How wrong I was.

(Midwife 30)

Yes that's what I mean, yes, that it happens somewhere else or to someone else or bad managing or bad communicating or caring scenarios or not in their unit. It happens up the road but it doesn't happen to us. Yes, I think that's a lot of the problem.

(Midwife 14)

There appears to be a defensive system operating, which is intended to protect from this unacceptable reality. The problem of what is effectively a form of occupational denial means that the midwife is not only unable to contemplate the possibility of a maternal death, but she is also unable to prepare herself for that possibility. That such preparation is feasible was fervently denied by some informants:

> RM: Others might like to prepare themselves as far as you're able to.
> MIDWIFE: Oh, I don't think you can, can you? How can you for such a. . . . You just don't know how you'd feel, y'know, until it happens.
>
> (Midwife 16)

> You can't prepare yourself in some ways for it. I mean when we were doing the supervisors course, they asked what would really worry you as a supervisor of midwives. And we all said 'A maternal death'.
>
> (Midwife 18)

Thus, the paradox between the expectations of midwifery and the reality became disconcertingly clear. This reality also manifested itself in the third major theme which emerged. This theme comprised the relationship between the midwife's professional experience and her personal life. The most impersonal aspect of this theme was the effect on the midwife's career and then her grief and attendance at the funeral. The most personal aspect, though, is the midwife's identification with the woman's experience and with those near at the time of her death. This identification, because of the 'grey-ing' of the midwifery profession, is likely to be with the mother of the woman who dies:

> I felt absolutely devastated. This is partly because my own daughter is the same age as she was. I feel that if she ever gets pregnant I'll be one worried person [nervous laugh].
>
> (Midwife 21)

These data lead to consideration of coping mechanisms in the event of a tragedy such as maternal death and the preparation and care for the largely female occupational group (Cudmore, 1996; Rose *et al.*, 2003).

The role of the supervisor

In the same way as the role of the midwife Manager has been shown to be important in the care of the grieving mother (please see Chapter 10), the role of the Supervisor of Midwives has been shown to matter in the context of the death of a mother (Mander, 1999c). Although the role of the Manager is clearly different from that of the Supervisor of Midwives (Stapleton *et al.*, 1998) this distinction has not always been well understood, and this may have applied to many of the midwives in my study of the midwife's experience of caring for a mother who dies.

The Supervisors described how they felt about the trauma of a maternal death, although in a way it was different from the experience of the clinical midwives. In spite of this, though, some Supervisors understood where their priorities lay:

> After all we did have a death before – one of the other Supervisors was involved – another woman who had a stillbirth and then she bled and she died on the unit. And the Supervisor said that she found that quite traumatic and she went off. She took three or four days off. She said 'I can't cope with this.' And at the time I thought that is our job really to be there with the midwives. It's important that we're there to support the midwives. I was quite conscious of the need for me to be there for the staff.
>
> (Midwife 18)

Some of the midwives mentioned instances of the Supervisor being supportive:

> We were contacted by our named Supervisor. How it happened was that there was a Supervisor on that evening when the death occurred and so she took the lead. My personal Supervisor is actually a community midwife manager. She operates an open door policy and she'd be there for me. She's really excellent. They might see you in the corridor and ask you if you're all right, things like that.
>
> (Midwife 14)

For some Supervisors, though, the system did not work so well, especially when the Supervisor expected her manager to be there for her:

> I rushed into my own office and burst into tears. You know, I felt better after that because people were crying but I sort of felt well I've got to keep going. I'm the Supervisor. I mustn't break down. Then I went downstairs to see my boss. The assistant head of midwifery was there. She was very, very supportive. I was able to tell her that I'd had a dreadful – an awful – night. My boss was just coming back from holiday and it always seems as if something happens when she's away – it always does. And I sort of walked in – and I don't know whether it was the fact that she'd just got back from holiday or what but she said 'Oh, God! Now what's happened?' Y'know, but her whole attitude was 'It's OK, now that she's in ICU.'
>
> (Midwife 18)

The reverse also occurred, when the midwife Manager expected the Supervisor to offer support:

> There was some criticism from my colleagues that I was being ineffective – that I was not being supportive enough. I suppose that this was my colleagues being competitive since my promotion to a managerial post.

It was very much a learning experience for all of us. I had to work out what was best for the future. I found out what was lacking and this was support. There was informal support. But a strong supportive framework was lacking. This reflects on midwifery Supervision – there is a need for best practice guidelines. We all too often find that support is offered, but it is not given. There is a need for a side-by-side relationship between the midwife and the Supervisor, which will provide support through emotional trauma, which is like an emotional eruption.

(Midwife 02)

It is apparent that the Manager and the Supervisor are aware of common areas in their respective roles, but are not certain how to resolve the overlap. This is apparent in the following example of the Supervisor not being supported:

And really through it all I felt that I gave support to everybody who I could. People – community midwives who came to the area to help us at the time – I wrote to everybody and thanked them all because I knew what a hard thing it was for everybody concerned. But personally I didn't feel that I got the appropriate amount of support from a more senior level. Not from my direct line manager anyway or from my Supervisor of Midwives. And that made it hard because I didn't feel that anybody ever said at any point 'thank you' for everything that you did, you did a good job or anything like that. It was only when I wrote down my statement about it that I realised myself what an onerous task I'd had. And my support for the other midwives, particularly who were directly involved, has gone on.

(Midwife 29)

It may be that, as well as emergency procedure protocols to deal with the events of the tragic incident, the roles of the personnel involved should be understood, to avoid such ongoing acrimony.

It is apparent from this research project that, in addition to the obvious disaster which a maternal death constitutes, there are a multiplicity of human issues which it brings with it. These personal and personnel issues need to be addressed if the staff providing care in these circumstances are not to be further and unnecessarily traumatised. It may be that strategies used to help staff in palliative care should be being used in the care of the dying mother (Mander and Haroldsdottir, 2002).

One of these human issues is the one that has been raised repeatedly in the Triennial Confidential Enquiries into Maternal Death (Lewis and Drife, 2004; Lewis *et al.*, 2001). This is the problem of ensuring effective teamwork in the event of life-threatening maternal illness, possibly leading to maternal death. The extent and effectiveness of teamworking does not attract any attention until its absence is observed in the context of the death of a mother. It may be suggested that this area of care deserves the attention of researchers in order to limit the effects of these disasters.

The safe motherhood initiative

It was an Inter-Agency Group which in 1987 focused the world's attention on the travesty which is maternal mortality. This group sponsored the conference in Nairobi which sought to raise world consciousness and begin to mobilise its resources. The aims which the Nairobi conference articulated, to reduce the number of maternal deaths by half by 2000, have proved naïvely optimistic. The extent of the shortfall is spelt out by Shiffman: 'it is not even certain that global levels of maternal mortality have declined in the past decade' (2003: 1198). This observation ignores the submerged majority of the iceberg of maternal morbidity.

The reason for this lack of success is less easy to explain. The fact that maternal mortality levels are a fraction in industrialised countries of what they are in developing countries may be taken to indicate that the problem is not insoluble. The knowledge exists among service users and providers in many developed countries to more or less match the maternity provision to the community's needs. It is providing appropriate and acceptable services in the developing countries which appears to present the major obstacle.

There is considerable diversity about the answer to this problem, to the extent that it gives the impression of being well-nigh intractable. An example is one of the basic priorities of the Safe Motherhood Initiative: ensuring trained and skilled attendance for the birth. While there is no question of the benefits of skilled attendants, the Safer Motherhood recommendation appears to be based on a correlation between lack of skilled attendants and high maternal mortality rates without having established causation. The research by Chapman (2003), though, shows the complexity of introducing skilled attendants. In her Mozambican example, cultural factors relating to the woman's vulnerability dissuade her from utilising such skilled assistance. In this way, cultural factors may impair progress at a practical level.

Other impediments may operate at different levels. Shiffman, in his analysis of the Indonesian situation (2003), demonstrates the fickle nature of the politicians' agenda. He shows how maternal mortality was all too briefly at the forefront of the politicians' concerns. As so often happens, due to a range of competing demands for their attention, the politicians' interest in maternal mortality waned. In Indonesia, though, quite serendipitously the spark of interest was rekindled through the publication of disconcerting mortality statistics in 1994. This resulted in the re-prioritisation of this issue and a new 'flurry of safe motherhood activity' (2003: 1202). In this way, the Indonesian situation was reinvigorated and rendered more effective.

Shiffman's (2003) analysis is useful, if only because it provides an indication of the complexity of the problem of maternal mortality. Recognition of this complexity is largely lacking in much of the Safe Motherhood literature.

All too often this problem is regarded as a single issue matter. This may be because a problem of these dimensions must be broken down into its constituent parts if it is to be rendered manageable. In spite of this, the impression remains that the various agencies involved are strenuously pursuing their own agendas with little regard for the issues which do not fit. For example, Thompson (1999) regards the problem as one of human rights, whereas in the same publication Thomson (1999) considers the main issue as international poverty. Fransen (2003) examines maternal mortality in terms of inequalities in education, finance and health provision. Thompson (2003) addresses the problem in personal terms and in terms of the role of the midwife. The solution for Maine and Rosenfield (1999) is found simply in the provision of medical treatment.

While all of these authorities may be correct as far as they go, they do not realise that they are not going far enough. It must be recognised that in the matter of maternal mortality there are many sensitive areas which constitute 'elephant traps' and of which agencies, if they are to be effective, must steer clear. To suggest that maternal mortality is a gender issue may result in labelling as feminist. In the same way, raising issues of women's rights may alienate certain fundamentalist persuasions. If maternal mortality is regarded as a family planning matter, certain religious groups will exclude themselves. If the problems of unsafe abortion are being addressed, the anti-choice/pro-life lobby becomes detached.

The question asked by Maine and Rosenfield (1999) is one that needs a more comprehensive answer than the medical solution which they provide: 'The Safe Motherhood Initiative: why has it stalled?' The answer to the question of maternal mortality is not the simple solution or the single issue beloved of the media, or the 'quick fix' which politicians need if they are to be re-elected. The answer must lie in the realm of culture change. Thus, many aspects of women's control over their lives need to be addressed, together with the education of men. Once safe motherhood is accepted as a long-term challenge which requires serious collaborative commitment at the highest level, there may be a chance of beginning to resolve the 'obscenity of maternal mortality' (Thomson, 2003).

Conclusion

In this chapter I have attempted to move maternal death away from the medical and epidemiological corner to which it has been relegated. I have sought to bring it into the arena of culture, care and grief. In order to do this, I have introduced some personal and political aspects. I have also indicated certain areas in which research is still very much needed.

10 Staff reactions and support

Observing their reactions to the loss of a baby, a psychiatrist described how staff are 'flung apart' by such a loss (Bourne, 1979). In this chapter I look at how members of staff are or are not able to cope with the experience of being 'flung apart' and the solutions which have been suggested to help them.

The relevance of Bourne's observation becomes clear in Curtis's oral history account of midwives attending the birth of a stillborn baby (2000). The midwife informants who began their practice between 1959 and 1968 recounted the practice of quickly removing the baby. This has become known as the 'rugby pass approach': 'once it was delivered and it was dead it was just sort of wrapped up and put away' (2000: 528). The rationale for this hasty removal was founded on the then widespread misunderstanding of the grieving process and our misplaced desire to protect the mother from further unnecessary anguish. This misunderstanding is implicit in the subsequent comments by Bourne in which, focusing on our medical colleagues, he reports the lack of research and literature relating to perinatal death. His own earlier research had identified the difficulty that some medical practitioners face when a baby dies, as evidenced by the inability of general practitioners to recall even basic factual information, such as the names of families in which a baby has died (Bourne, 1968).

The reason for the significance of the reaction of the member of staff is spelt out by Osterweis et al. (1984). Adopting an institutional approach, they suggest that health care personnel cannot be expected to provide optimal care and support for the dying and the grieving, unless allowance is made for both their personal or family tensions and their occupational, especially grief-related, problems. The need for us as carers to be emotionally secure has also been raised in more general situations. For example, in a more purely stress-related context, Cole suggests that 'in order to have healthy patients you need to have healthy staff' (1993). Thus, it may be that emotional health is a fundamental requirement for those who provide care in potentially stressful situations.

The reasons why members of staff may experience difficulty in coping with perinatal death are threefold. First, on a personal level, we find the death of a baby shocking because it is untimely or unnatural, that is, outwith the normal cycle of birth, life and death (McHaffie, 2001: 6). Although as daughters and sons we know that we are likely to grieve the death of our parents, parents do not expect to have to mourn the death of their children. Perhaps because of this untimeliness, the loss of a baby raises many deeply felt, long-hidden and perhaps unrecognised emotions, which may be associated with our memories and anticipations of past and future intimate losses.

Second, on a professional level, the loss of a baby represents a failure in our abilities as carers to perform that function which our chosen occupation requires of us – assisting with the birth of healthy babies. The fact that perinatal death has been entitled 'the ultimate defeat' (Queenan, 1978) indicates the difficulty which some may encounter in assisting with the care of a baby who is not alive and healthy. This perception of failure in care gives rise to negative feelings among professionals, which have been identified by Stack (1982) in terms of helplessness, defeat, guilt, resentment and failure. The prospect of the death of a baby, and the negative feelings arising from it, may result in the desire to avoid that death at any cost (Peppers and Knapp, 1982). This avoidance develops into a confrontation, in which carers may have to face the 'ultimate defeat' mentioned already.

Third, in terms of our learning, we tend to practise and become more skilled in doing those things in which we have been trained or in which we have experience; the corollary of this is that, if we have not been trained or have not become experienced in handling a particular situation, we will not only not learn about it, but we may seek to avoid situations exposing our deficiency and the anxiety it engenders. Buckman (2000) applies this rationale to the care of the dying adult, but it is not difficult to find similarities with our care for a grieving mother. He concludes that areas that are 'out of bounds' early in our careers remain that way throughout our working lives. We may surmise that this sequence may continue indefinitely on a cyclical basis if the insecurity and anxiety which these 'no-go' areas engender are passed on to future generations of carers for whose education we are responsible.

It is clear that, for any or all of these reasons, we may find ourselves fundamentally, and possibly disconcertingly deeply, affected when a baby is lost. Whether we are able to recognise in ourselves the extent to which we are personally affected by such a loss is less clear. The need to identify and acknowledge the personal implications of a death is fundamental to being able to care effectively for those who are dying and grieving. Without these personal precursors, it may be that a range of variably harmful consequences ensue.

The staff's personal reactions may result in the need for greater openness, which still applies to some midwives and their colleagues. In the research which I have mentioned already (Mander, 1995b), I found that the concept of professionalism still held sway with some midwives. This emerged in what 'Bessie' told me when I asked her about sharing tears with a grieving mother:

> There are two schools of thought about it. First, there is the old school which says that you must retain your professional thing quite intact. The second view is that you grieve with the woman. I think that it really depends on the midwife and the woman. I am quite happy to hold her hand or to put my arm around her shoulder, but I think you need to stay a professional.

Other health care providers have found a similar difficulty in coping with the grieving mother or couple:

> It was the way [the registrar] came in several times and he just stared at us ... didn't say nothing. ... I don't know whether he couldn't handle it. . . . He just stared at us. Sort of to say, 'There's nothing I can really do much'.
>
> (Moulder, 1998: 126)

That some recognition is emerging appears in a later informant's comment:

> I wish there was something that you could give [the grieving mother] in the way of support. But I don't know whether that's possible really and, I don't know, perhaps the doctor isn't the right person to become involved.
>
> (Moulder, 1998: 126)

This need for greater openness may relate not only to our ability to provide care, but also to our experience of providing that care. In a caring situation it might be suggested that experiencing the actual pain of caring for a grieving mother is part of the caring experience, and the pain of caring may help us to care more effectively. In the same way as grief provides the bereaved person with opportunities for personal growth, caring for a grieving mother may facilitate personal and professional growth and real interaction. Thus, teaching of health care providers in general and midwives in particular needs to focus on the reality of care in loss, including teaching about genuine engagement rather than superficial attitudes as exemplified in the 'rugger pass' approach.

Stress

It seems self-evident that the reasons why staff experience difficulty are also reasons likely to engender stress in care providers. Unfortunately, as Carlisle and colleagues found in 1994 and still applies, stress among midwives has been subjected to minimal research attention. More typically, the stress experienced by nurses has been applied to the maternity setting, such as nurses caring for dying adults in a palliative care setting (Kirstjanson *et al.*, 2001). These nurses' stress was found to be aggravated by their inability to prevent the more unsettling deaths.

The extent to which caring for a grieving mother is stressful for us as carers emerged during my research (Mander, 1995b). In the course of her interview, Kay explained that, for midwives, the stress of grief is likely to be superimposed on the, usually tolerable, stress level associated with conscientious practice:

KAY: It's a difficult situation. . . . It's a situation of grief; anybody who's trained as a nurse will tell you that working with people who are dying is a very stressful occupation. Midwifery per se – delivering healthy babies – is stressful 'cos there's always the worry of 'I hope everything's all right'.

The way in which Kay talked about 'stress' reflects the current general usage of this word. We tend to perceive stress as a uniformly negative phenomenon, arising from a range of unpleasant experiences to which we are subjected (Conduit, 1995). This perception of the invariably negative nature of stress was called into question by the work of Selye (1956), when he looked at stress in physiological terms and concluded that it is a universal adaptive response. He named this response the General Adaptation Syndrome, or 'GAS'. Although many of our ideas about stress have moved on since Selye undertook his work, we should give him credit for his emphasis on the likelihood of stress being a response to a range of possibly threatening, challenging or even enjoyable stimuli (Selye, 1980).

Selye's account of the nature of stress neglected the significance of individual factors, such as emotional and physiological characteristics, in the interpretation of stress. The interactionist explanation of stress is now more generally accepted (Lazarus, 1976), which interprets stress as the interaction of the relevant features of the environment with the person who is perceiving the situation.

The interactionist view recognises that different people interpret the same situation as threatening, challenging or enjoyable to differing extents. The interpretation of the same person may also differ, possibly over time, associated with learning about a situation or possibly due to other factors which make the person more or less vulnerable. A crucial feature of the interactionist view of stress is the significance of the person's interpretation of the situation in which they find themselves. We need to be wary of belittling another person's perception of the stress they experience – as with certain other phenomena we should accept that it is what the person experiencing it says it is.

The stress which is experienced by those staff involved in the loss of a baby is a topic which has been widely neglected. The reaction of the nurse caring for an adult who is dying has been studied in North America and the reactions of student nurses have been studied in the UK (Bailey and Clarke, 1991). These authors suggest that the response of the nurse to the death of a patient is variable and includes positive as well as negative elements. The positive aspects include feelings of the nurse having done her best for the patient or having helped the relatives in the most appropriate way. The less positive aspects may include any of the many emotions which we face when a person dies.

Bailey and Clarke (1991) discuss the relative merits of the nurse being older and/or more experienced in helping her to perceive death and dying as less negatively stressful. In her research, Hockley (1989) found that experience made little difference to the degree of anxiety the nurse feels when caring for a dying adult, but the focus of that anxiety does differ. Those nurses with less experience tend to be more concerned about controlling their own emotions, whereas more experienced nurses worry about their responsibility to the patient and the relatives. Judging the value of age and experience in coping with perinatal death is even harder. This is because it is complicated by, first, the way in which we as carers in the maternity area identify strongly with those for whom we care and, second, the not insignificant input of personal childbearing experience into our care (Mander, 1992b).

Factors contributing to stress

Certain features, the midwives in my recent study told me, exacerbated their perception of stress associated with the loss of a baby. These features increased their vulnerability and may have compromised the care they were able to provide for the grieving mother.

Difficulty

The midwives described the challenge which caring for a grieving mother presents; this relates to the threefold difficulties which I have mentioned already. Although learning about a situation may lower the stress which it engenders, Hattie, a midwife with many years' experience, told me how caring for this mother did not become easier for her:

HATTIE: No matter how many of these mothers you deal with, it's always a very difficult situation. It's not easy having to cope with your own emotions and to care for the mother as well.

Part of this difficulty may be due to the problems which we as carers face in recognising our own emotions, which is clearly a prerequisite if we are to provide effective care through good communication:

BETTY: It's hard for them and it's hard for us to talk about the death, so we have to work hard to build up a relationship in which they can express their feelings.

Occasionally the non-verbal messages given by the midwife warned me that her difficulties with even discussing the grieving mother were too sensitive for me to probe any further:

FLORRIE: I think it is a personal thing with me. It is not something I would like to have to deal with. I would find it quite difficult.

A perceptive comment by Queeny about the difficulty of staff in caring for the grieving mother was accompanied by a facial expression which suggested that she was aware that what she was saying might not be generally acceptable:

QUEENY: I can't help feeling that sometimes the staff have difficulty caring for this woman and this may be part of the reason for her getting home so soon.

Queeny's comment endorses my earlier suggestion that our difficulties in caring for the grieving mother may be associated with our sense of failure and may lead to avoidance of further potentially painful encounters. The problems which we encounter when communicating with dying people and their relatives are well known. Fanny spelt out the feelings shared by the midwives I interviewed:

FANNY: I find a lot of times it's very difficult to know what to say to them. Obviously, you don't want to upset them any more than they already are. Sometimes it's difficult to know whether they want to talk about it or whether they don't want to talk about it. I think that's very difficult. But they need to talk.

Midwives told me how, ordinarily, they use the prospect of the mother having a healthy baby to encourage her during her labour. Being unable to use this form of encouragement was sadly missed and caused the midwife to experience difficulty which would aggravate any pre-existing stress:

IRENE: Usually when I'm caring for women in labour, I take a very positive approach and tell them that their contractions are bringing them nearer to the birth of the baby . . . you can't say this and so it is difficult to encourage her, so it has to be more a case of 'one pain at a time'.

Being aware that she 'can't say' certain things acts as a further source of stress with which the midwife has to cope.

Those midwives who work primarily in the community encounter difficulties which might be solved relatively simply, such as the postnatal check which is usually undertaken in the mother's home. Grieving parents were said to have assumed that the midwife is there to examine the baby; this apparent error in care may cause further unhappiness if the parents are not warned that the midwife will be coming to visit the mother.

Although some of the difficulties we encounter when caring for grieving parents are fundamentally profound, others are merely organisational matters which are easily solved or, preferably, prevented. These organisational matters emerged in the study by Carlisle and colleagues (1994).

Lack of a happy outcome

Some of the staff who work in the maternity area are first attracted to it because they expect it to be a 'happy' area in which to work. Medical writers are very much aware of the relative rarity of perinatal death and that this may be seen as a benefit. Bourne (1979) supports this view and states that the attraction of obstetrics is in its healthy orientation and the possibility of 'some legitimate retreat from death and disease'. He goes on to spell out the unsuitability of this mental stance for the, albeit rare, perinatal deaths, the unhealthy consequences and the potential for psychiatrists to contribute more constructively. Likewise, Peppers and Knapp (1982) describe the particular difficulty that physicians may have in dealing with death, requiring that it be avoided at all costs, going on to state that, for obstetricians and paediatricians, the acceptance of perinatal death may be especially challenging. This difficulty may be explained by the unrealistically high standards which medical staff may set themselves in their fight against perinatal deaths, resulting in the painful personal costs which have to be paid by the staff member. In their discussion of the prevalence of the death-denying culture which we inhabit, Zimmermann and Rodin (2004) recognise that this criticism applies at least equally to medical practitioners. It may be that nurses and midwives are ahead of their medical colleagues in their realisation that death and dying are fundamental aspects of human life and, as such, deserve as high a standard of care as any other.

The comments of Irene (above) indicate the way in which midwives perceive the need to behave in a different, perhaps less relaxed, way if the mother will be grieving not having her baby with her. The regret for the absence of the usual happy ending is apparent in a comment by Josie:

JOSIE: Whereas with the lady who had an intra-uterine death . . . you haven't got a happy outcome at the end of it. It is a *totally* different situation you've actually got to cope with.

Unpreparedness to care for a mother who is grieving the loss of a baby may cause difficulties, especially for those who come into maternity care anticipating that it will be invariably enjoyable.

The mother's anger

An aspect of the grief reaction which exemplifies the contrast with the usual happy outcome and with which carers find particular difficulty in coping is anger. Although her anger is largely unfocused, for those of us who are with the mother on a twenty-four-hour basis, we will inevitably be on the receiving end of these powerful emotions:

NANCY: Some people are really angry at first especially with hospital staff. They feel that maybe the hospital was at fault or whatever; then some people just feel angry. I think that's part of the grieving process. I think you've just got to wait till the anger subsides and accept it.

RM: D'you find that a bit hard to take?

NANCY: I suppose that it is difficult but you've got to realise that it's just part and parcel of the whole process and not hold it against anyone for feeling that.

As well as the possibility of perceiving her anger as a personal insult, we have to consider its effect on our ability to care for the mother. Ruby indicates that it may act as a barrier to communication and, hence, caring:

RUBY: The staff maybe resent that so much of the anger is directed towards them. They have to get over that barrier initially.

While recognising the difficulty, Ginnie indicates a mind set which helps her to work through the mother's superficial confrontational stance:

GINNIE: Well, I don't think you would be human if you didn't [find the anger hard to take]. But you've got to remember that it is not directed personally at you . . . y'know. I mean obviously this woman has had a very traumatic experience, so I don't really find it hard to take. As I say, you've got to get to know the woman; it's very important.

Getting to know the woman, in spite of the antagonistic facade which she presents, imposes heavy demands on the resources of those caring for her. It is necessary now to consider the nature and adequacy of those resources.

Limited resources

The care which we are able to provide for the grieving mother is constrained in a number of ways. The resources which we have at our disposal are finite, unlike the demands, which often appear infinite. In considering the limitations on what we are able to offer the grieving mother, I focus, first, on the personal factors which are integral to us as carers and, second, on the organisational or more external facilities.

Personal factors

The midwives I interviewed were aware of their own shortcomings and were far from complacent about their care:

KAY: You just don't know what to tell a mother that's losing her baby or giving birth to a baby that well may not live.

The midwives told me that part of their concern related to their limited knowledge, which they attributed to inexperience due to the infrequency with which they encounter perinatal loss:

TRUDY: There is a great danger that the parents may be given incorrect information about some aspect, particularly of the procedures involved. This is probably because it is such an infrequent experience for each midwife and so she may not have very much knowledge about it.

Although our minds may inevitably turn first to the problems faced by staff in the labour ward, those who work with mothers postnatally face similar difficulties:

NELLIE: I can't say that I was particularly well prepared to cope. . . . I'd never actually met a mother who'd lost her baby before. . . . I came on [duty] and was told there was a mother who'd had a stillbirth and I remember the first time I went in to see her and I thought I've got to see to this woman and I've got nothing to say to this woman. There is nothing I can say to this woman to help her. How do I cope with her and support her?

Wendy spelt out the feelings of inadequacy to which Nellie was referring:

WENDY: We're just not sure what to say in a situation such as that and we are frightened to put our foot in it and we're frightened of the reaction of the mum. [The midwife's] emotions are so fraught at these times, nervous, in case we say the wrong thing or do the wrong thing.

The midwives told me of how they thought that these feelings of inadequacy might be remedied:

EFFIE: I think at that time, having looked after somebody like that . . . your own feelings of inadequacy at that time, you felt you wanted to go and read just to see if there was anything – what other views there were and what you should do in that situation.
FLORRIE: The other thing I would say is that we as midwives should have some special counselling or it should be necessary for all of us to attend some type of course, seminar or whatever so we are better equipped to deal

with it. 'Cos until I came to this [labour] ward about three months ago I had never come across these women.

Their lack of experience in caring for a grieving mother may be partly due to the practice in some units of only particular staff being involved. Clearly the expertise of the bereavement counsellor is helpful to the grieving mother, but other staff find that their own anxieties and feelings of inadequacy are aggravated:

QUEENY: I find, and I'm sure a lot of other midwives do, difficulty in treating this lady. This is because it's the Nursing Officer who counsels her and so the midwives don't get much opportunity to talk to her.

Organisational factors

In her research, Hockley (1989) found that nurses caring for adults who were dying experienced stress when they were unable, due to lack of time, to provide the care which they knew to be necessary. In the same way the need to be able to spend time being available to the grieving mother caused many midwives to be acutely conscious of the pressures on their working time.

DEIDRE: In the [. . .] wards I think it is a bit more difficult because you have people coming up after having a stillbirth and often you have several patients to look after or you are in charge and you don't have a lot of time to spend with them, or not enough time.

This in turn made them realise the deficiencies in their care:

NELLIE: We try our best to give them as much time to talk to us as possible. But I feel that really that isn't as good as we should be doing. We should be able to say I'm going to be here for an hour so; let's sit down and talk about it. What is really needed is more time to allow us to talk to these mothers and provide reassurance about the things that worry them. How we achieve this is not quite so easy. Perhaps we need more staff, or it may be that we could do with less patients.

The difficulties the midwives faced in prioritising their work became overwhelmingly clear. Problems of resources were also recognised as outwith both the midwife's province and the health service:

GINNIE: I sometimes feel like banging my head off the wall. I can't give them enough support. My anger is with myself and with others, such as the social work departments – they don't have enough resources to care as much as these mothers need. Some of them are quite comfortably off while others have got nothing. I often feel frustrated that I am unable to do more for them. All these cutbacks mean that the mothers aren't getting so many milk tokens and because the milk firms have stopped giving out samples we can't even help them out with those any more.

The frustration clearly articulated by Ginnie was apparent in Kay's comments about the organisational resources available to support her:

KAY: It's very stressful and I think senior midwives, they often push someone in who they think can cope with the situation and leave them to it, without really realising that that midwife needs support as well. It's not easy. It's stressful. We're not talking about a normal day's work – it's not a normal day's work – this happens maybe once every six months to every midwife if they're very unfortunate, maybe less often. So I think they need support. I think very often you're just left to get on with it – just by sheer workload, y'know, of a unit. And I think senior midwives have got to realise that that person has got to get some TLC as well.

Kay recognises that managers should make allowance for our need for 'tender loving care' (TLC), reminding us of the manager's responsibility for the working environment. This environment should be conducive to the provision of an optimal standard of care as well as being safe, that is not harmful, for staff. The work of Carlisle and her colleagues (1994) suggests that midwives' working environment may not comply with the latter standard in that their working environment is more likely to engender stress than that in which nurses practise. That Carlisle and colleagues' slightly dated findings are still relevant is endorsed by the work of Jowett (2003). The stress-related features of the maternity environment include, according to Carlisle and colleagues, discontinuity of care, lack of engagement with individual women, lack of support and limited autonomy. It may be that what Carlisle and colleagues unwittingly identified is the paradox between midwives' high expectations of autonomy and fulfilment and their disappointment with working in NHS institutions. As a nurse, Carlisle may be unaware of the level of the aspirations which new midwives bring with them and the contrast between those aspirations and the reality of providing a maternity service.

Kay's reference to 'TLC' resonates with Niven's thoughts about the multiplicity of demands on health care professionals (1992). She compares the stress experienced by a new mother in caring for and caring about her new baby with the stress that we may encounter when responding to the needs of the mothers in our care, as well as the demands of our lives outside our work. Although these non-work activities may be stressful in a negative sense, they may also provide us with an opportunity to 'recharge our batteries' and help us to get our work challenges into perspective. This brings us to consider how we, as members of staff, are helped to cope with the stress of these aspects of our work.

Factors helping to alleviate stress

So far in this chapter I have shown that the difficulties that we encounter when a mother is grieving are due to the way in which factors within ourselves interact with factors in the environment. These difficulties were described by the midwives in my recent study in terms of 'stress' which they, like many others, perceived entirely negatively. Stress may manifest itself in the early stages in the form of sickness absence or absenteeism or accidents or errors and in the later stages in what has become known as 'burnout' (Maslach, 1982; Hillhouse and Adler, 1997). We may regard sickness absence as a coping strategy, which probably equates in terms of helpfulness with those listed by Lazarus (1976) including denial, escape, displacement and intellectualisation. In this section we will be thinking about the more constructive and supportive methods which are used and have been suggested to adjust to stress generally (Mander, 2001c) and to the stress of caring for a grieving mother in particular.

There may be difficulty in either offering or accepting support to or from colleagues. Bond (1986) suggests that our own expectations and those of people near to us may prevent us from admitting our need for support. Additionally, an element of 'reaction formation' may be present, through which we act 'in the opposite direction to an impulse or desire which is being repressed' (Drever, 1964). We may find either or both of these mechanisms in action to conceal our vulnerability.

The largely adverse press which peer support has received in the nursing culture has been summarised by Sutherland as 'a pejorative term which is applied only to people who are considered weak' (Cole, 1993). This observation appears to be supported by the experience of Annie:

ANNIE: There can be situations where the support [from my colleagues] would
   be lacking. I think that it is isolated. I don't think it is a general rule . . .
   isolated incidences where support maybe wasn't there. I would say that
   all [this sounds terrible] – all the different kind of paperwork and everything, I would say you have a lot of help with that, but emotionally I
   wouldn't say that I have had particularly any help in that kind of way.

In spite of all these adverse observations, we can all call to mind occasions when we have found timely and effective support among our colleagues.

Peer support

Midwives' ability to support each other, as I have mentioned already, is variable (Kirkham, 1999). In terms of the limited provision of peer support, Stapleton and her colleagues (1998) show the painfully stark contrast between the support which midwives feel they should, and presumably do, provide for the childbearing woman, and the support which they make available for each other. It may be assumed that this extension of such supportive behaviour to colleagues may be so commonplace that it is taken for granted. This important and authoritative research project, however, suggests that this is far from the case: 'there was a painful contradiction between their need for support, and the fact that the culture of midwifery could not acknowledge, nor provide for that need' (Stapleton *et al.*, 1998: 142).

On the other hand, my research project on the midwife's experience of caring for a mother who dies (1999b; see Chapter 9) shows that in a comparable situation collegial support is able to be both timely and satisfying. In fact, the support provided on an informal basis by her midwife colleagues was the most highly valued of all sources of support for the midwife who had cared for a mother who died. This finding is comparable with the observation of the benefits of 'mutual support' (Stapleton *et al.*, 1998: 142) and 'fellow workers' support' (Munro *et al.*, 1998). The form which this support assumes may have been little more than a brief 'How's things?' when passing in a corridor. Alternatively, it may have been in the form of a few tears shared in the quiet of the staff coffee room.

This satisfying collegial support was not necessarily real. The potential for support or the perception of that support may have been sufficient. This often took the form of colleagues exchanging phone numbers with genuine encouragement to make contact if needed (Munro *et al.*, 1998; Metts *et al.*, 1994).

> And those of us who are kind of late 40s and have seen it before – we try really hard if there's a junior staff midwife involved to say 'Look, here's my home phone number . . .'
>
> (Midwife 13)

Occasionally, for a minority of midwives, this collegial support was not felt to be forthcoming. Such a lack of support applied to one of the midwives, who was so seriously affected by the experience that she became unwell and withdrew from midwifery practice for a while. It also applied to another midwife who had been temporarily thought to have been practising negligently: she felt unsupported to the point of ostracism for the few days while the standard of her practice was being seriously questioned:

> First of all there was no support for me, but when it was found that I was not to blame all the people around were more supportive of me. The only support I had was the head nurse, who was supportive throughout – right from the start and also my two close friends. The memory of it has stayed there ever since and it always will be with me.
>
> (Midwife 28)

For midwives such as Midwife 28, where collegial support was unforthcoming, the occupational and social isolation which the midwife inevitably seems to feel as a result of the death of a mother was seriously aggravated (Sarason *et al.*, 1994; Hingley and Marks, 1991).

> But I found it quite an isolating situation. Because maternal death isn't something that happens every day, thank the Lord, and I found it isolating because people would come to me and say 'I don't know what to say to you because this hasn't happened to me and I don't know how you're feeling' and a lot of people actually wrote that down.
>
> (Midwife 12)

A form of support which emerged as crucially valuable was that which arose out of the shared experience of the midwives who had actually been present when the mother died. Usually this shared experience related to the death of one particular woman, but for some midwives it applied to events which may have been separated by years and continents.

> MIDWIFE: I think the midwife who was the senior midwife, she was very understanding. Probably because she'd been there for many years but she's retired now. She'd had a maternal death about five years previously and so she had experienced what I was going through.
> RM: Her experience equated with yours?
> MIDWIFE: Yes. Yes. And she spent a great deal of time with me.
>
> (Midwife 22)

The midwife who found the support of another who had had a similar experience appreciated the insights which they were able to share together. This need to share the experience applied more particularly to those who may have cared for one mother around the time of her death. Thus, the sharing of the experience of loss emerged as highly supportive to the midwife or midwives who was or were seeking to recover from the death of a mother.

> Just after her death I had a strong feeling of wanting to be more with the colleagues who were there at the time. . . . After the shift finished I found that I wanted to be with my colleagues who had shared that experience. There was a need for us to be together. We just sat there and did not do anything. There was some tea made, but it did not get poured. We did not want to leave. It was really a case of just being together. We were all very shocked and quiet. The affected staff were keeping close. Our feelings were such that could not be shared with others. The feelings were too raw to share. The affected group kept close together
>
> (Midwife 04)

I found it a lot easier to talk to midwives and to take their sympathy if they'd either been there on the day it happened and worked with me through that day or worked with [the woman] the two or three days before. I found it much more difficult to talk to people who did not even know [the woman] even though they were being really good and trying to be very supportive as well, in the best way that they knew how.

(Midwife 12)

This 'closed circle' of midwives who had shared the experience was obviously very supportive to those who were part of it, but for some midwives being or not being involved in a particular incident became divisive. These divisions emerged in the form of criticism of those who were involved, as reported to me by a non-clinical midwife who had been closely involved with the death of a mother and who had sought to deal with these divisions in the staff of the maternity unit.

after it had happened some of the other midwives in the unit who weren't there on [duty] that Sunday, or the Monday, y'know, were passing comments. 'Oh well yes of course she was in pain or they should've done so and so' . . . or whatever or 'Yes, well, I know [the family] and they are going to complain.' And that was quite hurtful. I said 'You weren't there at the time, you don't know what was happening and if you can't say anything constructive . . .'

(Midwife 18)

Managers' support

As the words of Midwife 18 (above) show, the midwife manager has an important role to play in both providing and facilitating support for vulnerable staff members, including both those affected by the death of a mother and those caring for a grieving mother. The manager's role encompasses both her expectations of her staff being able to cope and the provision of adequate human resources; adequacy refers to the appropriate number of staff and those with the relevant skills. The need for the manager at the level of the ward or other clinical area to be aware of any emotional vulnerability in any of her staff is discussed in Chapter 11.

In her account of one clinical area in a major maternity unit, Foster emphasises the role of the manager in providing effective support for staff in situations of loss (1996). She argues that the midwifery manager needs to understand and recognise the stressors under which midwifery and other staff provide care. Such understanding, she proposes, influences the working environment for the better and, indirectly, the care which is offered. In her account of managing nursing in a palliative care setting, Lugton (1989) shows how senior staff are encouraged to serve as role models, possibly by encouraging other staff to accompany them when they are speaking with people who are dying or grieving. Lugton also highlights the role of managers in creating an organisationally secure environment, meaning that staff understand the extent and limits of their own and each other's roles and are able to function within them. This is likely to prevent conflicts between staff, which may give rise to confusion and uncertainty among those for whom they care.

We should also recognise the ability of a manager to establish the kind of therapeutic milieu in which clinical nurses and midwives are able to provide genuinely helpful care for people who are grieving. In one maternity unit, I was told repeatedly about the admirable management skills of a midwife whose job was threatened due to the recent closure of a clinical area:

YOLANDY: We had a very good senior midwife up there. She really helped us a lot and helped us to cope a lot.

In view of their overwhelming perception of working under pressure, the need for managerial action to provide adequate numbers of appropriately skilled staff becomes even more important:

MOLLY: Spending enough time listening to the mother can be difficult in these big wards. When you have twenty-eight or thirty-two patients in the ward it can be, and you only have four staff.

Some of the midwives told me how they made decisions about prioritising their own work and Gay recounted how she sought support from midwives in another area:

GAY: Well, that lady that had the stillbirth, we were busy that day but I just stayed with her. Y'know, and the rest of the patients I dealt with when the other staff came on. Y'know? I'm just going from that one experience that I had. I really stayed with her until she went down to the labour ward. She got priority. Yeah. And you can always ring to the labour ward – if they're quiet – for help, which is quite good in this unit. If the place is quiet they'll come up and give you a helping hand.

I have been considering the role of the manager in providing support for individual midwives who feel negatively stressed by the demands of their work and the limited resources available to them. These short-term managerial interventions provide much-needed on-the-spot support, but they have to be reinforced by more long-term, ongoing support which, in the same way, is likely to result from management innovation.

Support and other interventions

In this section I look at the more formal organisation of support for staff caring for the mother who is grieving. These interventions have been classified using a public health orientation according to their relationship with the onset of symptoms of stress (Van Wyk *et al.*, 2004; Reynolds, 1997). This categorisation begins with primary prevention, which aims to prevent the onset of problems by removing causative factors in the individual's working environment. Examples would include changing adverse job characteristics or increasing the individual's autonomy and control over their work.

Secondary prevention in a public health sense seeks to reduce the severity and/or duration of health problems in order to reduce the risk of them becoming chronic or disabling. In the work setting, secondary intervention would include the identification of employees who are considered as being at risk of stress-related health problems and intervening to prevent their deterioration. The interventions would comprise educational opportunities to help these employees to cope more healthily with the challenges which their work imposes.

Tertiary interventions in public health refer to the treatment of existing health problems to either cure the condition or limit its damage. In the work place, tertiary interventions would include debriefing, rehabilitation, medical treatment or psychotherapy or counselling.

Support groups, which are regarded by Van Wyk (2004) as a form of secondary prevention, have attracted some interest in the maternity area. In Southampton a member of the midwifery teaching staff involved a psychiatrist in establishing an informal, interdisciplinary support group (Roch, 1987). The group welcomed visitors, such as representatives from SANDS and other lay support groups and bereaved mothers, to contribute. The author emphasises the non-hierarchical nature of this group. This lack of a hierarchical structure is clearly crucial if a support group is to provide the safe environment in which more reluctant colleagues are able to 'open up'. The organisers deserve credit for breaking through the hierarchical barriers, although unfortunately we are not told how this remarkable feat was achieved, as this structure is all too pervasive in midwifery. Similarly, the multidisciplinary nature of this group appears to be another of its strengths. The membership includes a range of personnel, some of whom are based outwith the hospital and outwith nursing and midwifery disciplines. The reluctance of medical staff to become involved is clearly a source of regret to the organisers and we may question the reason for such reluctance.

In Preston a support group with a different remit was established (Sherratt, 1987). Interaction between lay people and professional carers is a priority for this group; consciousness-raising features as a major element – 'the topic needed to be brought to the notice of the general public'. The support of members of staff appears to be secondary to providing information and help for grieving parents and those near to them. In spite of this, the passage of information is clearly a two-way exercise; this results in staff learning, from those who have actually experienced perinatal grief, of the most appropriate way to care.

An account of setting up a medical and nursing staff group in a NNU indicates some of the problems encountered (Bender and Swan-Parente, 1983). Non-attendance was initially a problem, which the organisers solved by negotiation with nursing managers about the provision of suitable accommodation and time. Non-attendance may have been due to the lack of a safe environment and anxiety about the maintenance of personal defence systems. A generally acceptable format eventually evolved, in which staff built on known case histories.

In the context of establishing a terminal care support team, Dunlop and Hockley (1990) explore the necessity for and pitfalls of organising an ongoing multidisciplinary support group. They describe how the honeymoon period for the group was ended by the realisation of the actuality of the task and mismatches between needs and skills. The impact of death shocked some group members' as did the perception of lack of support from 'uncooperative doctors, unfeeling nurses and ungrateful patients'. Gradually personal and professional conflicts within the group became evident and the tendency to suppress them was overcome. Dunlop and Hockley refer to the group coping mechanism as 'chronic niceness', which was a short-term strategy to disguise the inevitable ill-feelings. Such feelings were discussed with group members other than the one directly involved, engendering factions and further disruption. Several months of 'chronic niceness' were necessary before the group felt safe enough with each other to respect others' strengths and to give them credit in a non-paternalistic way. These authors show us the value of group meetings for reflecting on difficult events. While working out 'what and who' made the situation difficult, allocating blame became a pitfall. Dunlop and Hockley go on to spell out the value of out-of-work group activities in helping to build relationships. Examples include pub lunches, theatre visits, picnics and other outings.

A major benefit of support groups lies in their ability to help us to work towards more realistic goals in our care of the dying. Our failure to meet unrealistic expectations may lead to withdrawal from involvement with patients, their relatives and colleagues. We may use a suitably safe and supportive group to ventilate our feelings of inadequacy. If we are able to deal with our negative feelings in this way, there are benefits not only for those for whom we care, but we, the carers, are likely to be more satisfied with the support we provide.

In advocating the introduction of peer support groups, Bond (1986) recognises the largely untapped ability of nurses to support each other. Referring to other non-peer support groups, she draws our attention to the willingness of 'group leaders', who tend to be male, to listen to the difficulties of a largely female caring staff. In contrast to this willingness to lead and listen, she highlights the reluctance of these leaders to relinquish their obviously responsible role by facilitating leadership skills within the group. Bond's accusation of such groups generating dependency among female colleagues may carry a familiar ring.

A problem which affects the organisation of support groups is the difficulty of making time. By definition, those of us who work in stressful environments are short of time. The question inevitably arises of how we, as individuals, are able to find time to give and receive support. Is it possible or appropriate for those of us who work in high-tech or otherwise stressful areas to assume that our employers will allow time for this form of recovery? The problem of time was raised by Bender and Swan-Parente (1983) and also by Roch (1987). The solution to which Roch and her colleagues resorted, was to arrange the group sessions to be held during the changeover of shifts, when traditionally there has been an overlap resulting in an approximately two-hour period with a double staff complement. Because this 'overlap' has been used for a range of activities which some consider inessential, such as meetings or teaching, the overlap has now disappeared. The result is that alternative time slots now have to be identified. The limited extent to which health authorities are prepared to make time available for support activities is raised by Cole (1993) in the context of group counselling. He shows us that the unpreparedness of employing authorities to allow support time reflects the limited priority given to staff welfare and perhaps, indirectly, to the support of those for whom we care.

It may be that Cole's suggestion of group counselling and support for those of us caring for people who are grieving is an ideal to aim for. Tschudin (1997) makes what may be a more realistic suggestion which comprises establishing services within an existing framework. She advocates that existing Occupational Health provision should extend its remit to include counselling services. She implicitly recognises the costs of providing this service when she states 'health authorities need to believe in the principle that prevention is better than cure'. Are staff support services another example of a phenomenon which is widely recommended, but rarely encountered?

A remembrance service

We all recognise the benefits of a funeral service for those who are grieving. I would like to question whether we, the caring staff, may appropriately use the funeral to express our grief, our support for the family and our support for each other. This concept emerged in my research project, initially in the context of the baptism of a stillborn baby whose mother requested that Gay, the midwife, perform this ceremony. I asked Gay about her reaction to this request:

GAY: I suppose that the service does help the staff a bit. You do . . . you probably do feel that you're doing something. I think the parents quite like it.

Ottily recounted to me her difficulty in attending the funeral of a baby:

OTTILY: I've never attended a baby's funeral. I suppose I've chickened out from going.

On the other hand Zy was able to recount her very different experience:

ZY: I go down to the hospital chapel with them . . . for the service. I think it is probably for both our sakes. Not just for the parents, I think for the staff's sake as well it makes a difference. I think of Jane, she is a staff midwife and not just newly qualified. She'd been so involved . . . with the lady who had the stillbirth and she had a talk with her. And we arranged a service and Jane came down to the service with us and afterwards she said, 'I feel a lot better.' We laughed at that so I think it really does the staff good as well as the parents themselves.

Our presence at the funeral requires great sensitivity. If the family is still experiencing anger or if some blame is being allocated, we may not be welcome at this quintessentially family event.

Summary

In this chapter I have considered the problems which we, as members of staff, may encounter when caring for a mother who is grieving the loss of her baby. Using data collected during my recent research, I have shown some of the reasons why we find this situation so difficult. I have then moved on to discuss the solutions which have been suggested to help us to cope better, in the hope that we will be able to provide more effective care.

11 Staff grieving and crying

The ways in which we, as members of staff, manifest our feelings in situations of loss vary hugely. The openness with which some of us feel comfortable reflects the behaviour which some others feel they ought to be able to offer; this in turn is balanced by a more 'stiff upper lip' approach for which others aim.

The manifestation of our reactions to loss may be changing as discussion of and personal responses to it become more open. In this chapter I show that change is happening, even since the work of Bourne (1979) who related how, even though staff are 'flung apart' by such a loss, some are able to show only 'aversion and silence'. To do this I draw on my research on the midwife's care of the mother who does not have her baby with her (Mander, 1995b) and other studies.

Emotional labour

Since the landmark work of the American researcher Arlie Hochschild in 1983, the way that employees manage their own emotions in order to achieve the aims of their employers has been the focus of considerable attention. Hochschild's original research examined the methods that two rather different groups of employees used to present the 'face' and thus maintain the emotional ambience sought by their employers. One of these groups has since become known as 'cabin crew'; the other group, with whose emotional labour we may be less well acquainted, were debt-collectors. Hochschild revealed the demanding nature of this form of work, which she described as 'emotional labour', although the term 'emotion work' may be used interchangeably (Bolton, 2000). Hochschild showed that cabin crew in particular are taught not to display their own genuine emotions in the interests of making passengers feel comfortable and confident. Thus, the concept of emotional labour has been defined as workers endeavouring to 'create and maintain a relationship, a mood, or a feeling' (Hochschild, 1983: 440).

Hochschild went on to differentiate the nature of what was effectively the play acting which employees were required to perform. 'Surface acting' involves only the worker's appearance in terms of her body language, when she is above all aware of the superficial nature of her behaviour. Infinitely more challenging, however, is the 'deep acting' which demands that the worker utilise her own experiences of emotional pain (1983: 36). Inevitably such a process taxes the worker's emotional reserves. In the two occupations which Hochschild studied, there was little altruistic rationale for burdening staff in this way.

Hochschild's ideas have found a ready and receptive audience in the health care system (James, 1992) and especially in nursing. It has been argued, though, that there has been a lack of attention to/recognition of emotion work in midwifery (Davies, 2001). Examples used to support Davies's argument include partnerships in care, the special nature of midwifery, the intimacy of midwifery work, working with women in pain and the division of labour. It may be surprising, in view of the all too obvious need for emotional labour at such times, that Davies does not mention the relevance of this concept in situations of loss. Similarly, I found no reference to emotional labour at times of loss or death in the nursing literature. It is necessary to question the reason for these situations being ignored. Perhaps the reason is that emotion work is all about acting, when the midwife faces very real emotions, as I discuss below and as I have shown elsewhere, albeit without using the title 'emotional labour' (Mander, 2000).

Crying as grieving

Crying emerged as an important issue in my study of the midwife's care (Mander, 1995b), having been the focus of some interest in the nursing media. Crying may be an example of one form of self-disclosure, which has attracted considerable attention in the mental health and, particularly, the psychoanalytic literature (Ashmore and Banks, 2001). It is a topic which has also emerged as an issue in human relations research (Pongruenphant and Tyson, 2000). In the present context, though, the issue relates to nurses' and midwives' concerns about whether it is appropriate to show and share grief through tears. A series of narratives included a number of accounts by nurses and midwives of their need and ability to share clients' and patients' grief by the use of touch, physical comfort and tears (Darbyshire, 1992). These narratives imply the reluctance of some of us to 'get involved' by showing our emotions. Each of the published narratives concluded on a positive note by indicating the benefits of sharing emotions for both the staff member and the client or patient (Diekelmann, 1992; Walker, 1992). In this chapter I consider how staff feel about those occasions when they may have cried and the factors which affect whether or not they cry. As well as using the limited literature on this topic, I draw on the comments made by midwives during my study (Mander, 1995b).

The reluctance of midwives to acknowledge that they have cried with a mother, implied in the Darbyshire narratives (1992), is apparent in Nancy's account of her care of a mother relinquishing her baby for adoption:

NANCY: I went with her to see her baby and she spoke to the baby and told her baby how she was sorry about giving him up and just explained that she couldn't look after him. It was really nice for someone who had denied it for so long . . .

RM: How did you manage?

NANCY: I was OK . . . and . . . no, I was crying actually.

The uncertainty many midwives feel about crying, which becomes more clear in the interviews described later, emerges in Marie's slightly defensive account of her more long-term relationship with the mother of a dying baby:

MARIE: There was a woman we had in . . . whose baby eventually died at three months. We became very close and very supportive to that mother and when her baby died we were all upset and we were crying along with the mother.

RM: Was that OK?

MARIE: We were crying, but that did not affect our ability to care. Even though we were upset we were still able to do our jobs. The day I don't shed a tear over a dead baby is the day I walk out the door of this place.

A survey which was undertaken in Sydney, Australia, is part of a larger cross-cultural programme looking closely at crying among certain groups of hospital staff (Wagner *et al.*, 1997). This study originated in the woeful anecdotes of medical students and practitioners, and the questionnaire which was applied was based on the authors' collections of these accounts. The questionnaire began by using a form of critical incident technique to probe the staff member's experience of crying in the hospital. This section was followed by others which probed attitudes and reactions to staff and patients crying. These included questions on who is and is not 'allowed' to cry, and the reactions and support available to crying staff.

Wagner and her colleagues sought a sample of nurses, medical practitioners and medical students, but encountered some difficulty, which may not be altogether surprising in view of the sensitivity of the topic. The sample selection appears to have been opportunistic, as the researcher walked into a ward and handed out the questionnaires to the staff 'on duty' (1997: 13). Medical students were given the questionnaires at university lectures. The response rate from medical practitioners was paltry, and mailings and reminders were necessary to produce the final response rate of 33 per cent (n=52). This may be compared with the unprompted rates of 58 per cent (n=103) from nurses and 99 per cent (n=101) from medical students. The gender balance among the nurses and students reflected the distribution in their groups. Among the medical practitioners, however, women were seriously overrepresented, constituting 57 per cent of the sample from an occupational group with only 29 per cent women. In view of this slightly strange sample, the results need to be interpreted with caution.

Table 11.1 Hospital staff reports of having cried at work (from Wagner *et al.*, 1997)

	Female respondents (%)	Male respondents (%)	Total (%)
Nurses	76/96 (79)	2/7 (28)	**78/103 (76)**
Medical Practitioners	18/27 (66)	11/25 (44)	**29/52 (55)**
Medical students	20/47 (43)	10/52 (19)	**30/99 (30)**
Total	**114/169 (67)**	**23/83 (28)**	**137/252 (54)**

The findings (Table 11.1) indicate that women health personnel are significantly more likely to have cried than their male equivalents. Female nurses are the most likely to have cried, whereas male medical students are least likely.

Unfortunately Wagner and her colleagues did not ask how comfortable or uncomfortable their respondents were with their tears. It may be that this comfort or lack of it among the three groups may be reflected in the researchers' ease of recruitment. My own data, however, show that we as staff experience ambivalence about showing emotions to those for whom we care. This is already clear and will become clearer as this chapter proceeds. That the mother welcomes the emotional contact with the midwife becomes apparent in the comment of a mother going through the process of relinquishing her son for adoption:

URSULA: After I came home . . . and the midwife came to see me, she was really lovely. When she was making her last visit she put her arm round me and gave me a big hug. It meant so much to me and it was so different from others I had met.

Crying and helping

The midwives I interviewed interpreted their preparedness to cry with a bereaved mother in terms of sharing emotions, or perhaps the potential for common feelings.

JOY: It's not out of the ordinary but I often find myself crying with them. This is because I hurt for them – it could be me.

POLLY: Yes, I have had tears in my eyes many a time with them. It is just a natural thing, I think. Just talking about it, it is natural to sympathise with them. I think it's human and what they need is the human touch.

FLORRIE: Well, y'know, everybody is human . . . what would be wrong, y'know, for somebody to feel a lump in their throat and start crying? I think that is quite acceptable and, and just to show that you have got feelings as well – and care.

The midwife's powerful sense of identification with the mother is obvious in these comments. Shared values and common experience are crucial in many aspects of midwives' care. They told me that they draw on many sources of knowledge and information when they are deciding on how to care, but the significance of their personal and occupational experience cannot be overstated (Mander, 1992b).

The naturalness and lack of deliberation when midwives cry seems to matter to those I interviewed. Even though it is spontaneous to behave in this open way, we don't always find it easy or comfortable.

FANNY: I personally can get quite emotional with the mother. Like if she was crying and talking, I could very easily join in and show that I also feel for her. That can help if she knows that you genuinely have sympathy with them and it's not just your job.

RM: How do you feel about that?

FANNY: I wouldn't say I feel comfortable, no. I have done it. I mean if I do genuinely feel if I was upset with someone I do genuinely feel that way. I wouldn't just do it to try to make them feel better. With someone losing their baby it's a very emotional thing for us, just as well as the mother. I certainly wouldn't be afraid to let someone know I felt sympathy and be upset at what had happened. I wouldn't be afraid to do that.

Fanny's comment introduces the spectre of the sense of failure which may be encountered by those of us who work in the maternity area, as well as the possibility of the reappearance of memories of other losses which may constitute our own 'unfinished business'.

Disapproving

As well as crying exposing the humanity and hence the vulnerability of us all, there are additional dimensions which we must consider when nurses and midwives contemplate crying. A narrative by a midwife recounting her care of a mother adjusting to her newborn son's terminal illness emphasises some of these dimensions: 'We cried together. I apologised for crying; I tried to say how unprofessional it was and that I was trained not to break down' (Walker, 1992). This quotation raises two of the significant issues in the context of the approval of staff crying. These are, first, the concept of 'professionalism' and, second, the education or training which prepares nurses and midwives to behave professionally. It is necessary to assume that the term 'professional' in this context is being used to mean efficient and distant as opposed to any other characteristics which we may attribute to professionals (Mander, 2004b). This form of behaviour was found to be the institutional norm in a care of the elderly setting (Costello, 2001). Darbyshire's commentary on Walker's narrative takes up the use of the term 'professional', suggesting that when used in this way the concept is so 'perverse' as to be unrelated to any form of human experience. In a nursing research project Cahill (1998) identified practices which firmly and inextricably linked 'professionalism' with 'distance'. The 'perversity' of such uses of the concept of professional behaviour does not prevent it from being widely used, perhaps as a coping mechanism (Menzies, 1969):

BESSIE: There are really two schools of thought about [staff crying]. First, there is the old school which says that you must retain your professional thing quite intact. The second view is that you grieve with the woman. I think that it really depends on the midwife and the woman. I am quite happy to hold her hand or to put my arm round her shoulder, but I think that you need to stay a professional.

The midwives were well aware that their behaviour in crying with grieving parents might engender disapproval:

EMILY: I know some people think that it is not professional, but I do some-times cry with the mother as this lets her see that we are human.
OTTILY: You can have a little cry . . . and nobody thinks any the less of you. You never used to be able to do that.
QUEENY: Yes, I have cried with a woman who has lost her baby. I think that you should be able to. After all it is a human thing to do and we are all human. I know that some people think that nurses should not cry, but I think that is wrong. We need to be able to share [her] sorrow.

The fear may exist that the perceived disapproval may actually materialise into overt criticism, so that, at a time when we expect helpful support from our colleagues, we may render ourselves even more vulnerable to hostile criticism:

QUEENY: There was a [mother] recently who lost her baby. I was very upset about it and so I cried with her. . . . I had to go to see the Nursing Officer about something and she said to me [loudly] 'What are you so upset for?' Some people don't approve.

The non-approval of nurses crying was highlighted by Dunlop and Hockley (1990) in the context of caring for dying adults. These authors discuss the benefits of maintaining a 'calm demeanor' as opposed to the suppression of 'strong emotions'. They show us the role of nurse training in creating the 'pull yourself together' ethos. Similarly, Walker's quotation leads me to question the appropriateness of systems of nursing and midwifery education which teach the student not only to cope effectively, but also to maintain a superficial appearance of efficiency:

KERRIE: but you know obviously you've got be very careful, keep your emotions in check . . . you feel very close to tears . . . you can feel the tears springing into your eyes but . . . y'know. I don't know why. I think it is something that is drummed into you during your training or that with upsetting things you've got to put on this brave face and, you know, just show the patient that you are coping and that you can't burst into tears.

Thus, as well as their own disapproval of their own behaviour, the midwives whom I interviewed were aware of others' disapproval. These findings reson-ate with the findings of Wagner and her colleagues (1997: 14) who asked respondents about the reaction of other staff and colleagues when they did cry. Although these researchers found that in all groups approximately half of those who cried were comforted, a similar proportion was not. Of those who were not comforted more than half were left alone. The remaining, admittedly small, proportion experienced an even more disconcerting out-come. These were the 21 per cent of medical students who were 'ridiculed, looked at with contempt or screamed at' (1997: 14). These unfortunate out-comes were also experienced by 9 per cent of medical practitioners and 2.5 per cent of nurses. It is a pity that the researchers indicate neither the occu-pational group nor the gender of those doing the ridiculing and screaming.

As with many aspects of human behaviour the cultural implications of crying need to be recognised. My sample of midwives was, in cultural terms, relatively homogeneous. The work by Wagner and colleagues (1997), how-ever, was the Australian component of a cross-cultural project, which has been replicated in Vienna, Austria (Barth *et al.*, 2004). The respondents in Austrian hospitals are generally marginally less likely than their Australian equivalents to 'allow' health workers to cry. Australian patients are only slightly more likely to be allowed to cry than their relatives, whereas in Austria this difference is much more clearly pronounced.

Although it is clear that midwives and other personnel consider that crying may sometimes be appropriate, they are both aware and wary of the possibil-ity of disapproval by other members of staff. Inevitably, the openness which sharing grief requires also renders the carer more vulnerable to criticism.

Crying real tears

While we may be generally approving of midwives crying with grieving par-ents, the implications of this approval for our midwifery practice may be less direct. For some of us there is no difficulty in putting our ideas about crying into practice:

JOY: For me it's so easy, so natural to put my arms around her and to cry with her. I often have.

For other midwives, such as Deidre, while approving of the idea of a midwife crying, there may be other factors preventing her from putting it into practice:

DEIDRE: If you feel like crying, I don't think you should stop yourself. I think some staff would probably not be able to cry in that situation because it wouldn't be comfortable. If that is the case – you have just got to be yourself. I haven't cried openly. I think I have had tears in my eyes and a lump in my throat, but I haven't actually sat down and cried.

RM: Is this because crying may affect your ability to care?

DEIDRE: I don't think that is true. I think if you are feeling like crying [and do] then you won't function any worse than if you bottle it up.

HATTIE: I think if she's feeling strong emotions, I don't see that there's any crime if she does [cry]. I know it was maybe the old idea that we should remain detached from parents. I think we've been part of something very dramatic in the woman's life. We can't alter that.

RM: Have you . . .?

HATTIE: Well, maybe not cried in front of the patient but I have felt very, very sad, maybe have gone out . . . felt very devastated if something has happened.

These quotations lead to the conclusion that some midwives may actually find crying with the grieving mother to be less acceptable and hence less likely to happen than the recommendations of openness would suggest.

Places to cry

Thus, a carer may feel uncomfortable sharing her tears with the grieving mother. She may still, however, consider it appropriate to give expression to her emotions in what she considers to be a safer environment. I consider now where this safer place to vent emotions may be.

The traditional place in a hospital ward for the disposal of waste is the sluice. In the sluice, or dirty utility room, used linen is collected for transfer to the laundry, we despatch human waste, such as bedpans' contents, and we bag used dressings and other material ready for incineration. Although I, and possibly others, have used the sluice for the secret disposal of emotional waste, including fury, frustration or sorrow, it was not mentioned by any of the midwives. Similarly, the linen cupboard, often publicised as the location of various unmentionable activities, was not suggested as a suitable place for crying.

Although Zy was initially unable to admit to crying with the parents, she eventually recalled that she had used the changing room for her tears and that this prepared her to share their grief more openly:

ZY: I have probably not been actually in tears . . . I tell a lie, there is one time I was absolutely . . . I had to adjourn into the changing room. I had got quite involved with one of the [mothers] and . . . and I just burst into tears and I felt better after it, but I think possibly we'd got more involved than we normally do . . . I had to go back and see them, and they said

'Oh, you've been crying.' So I had a chat with them, and a wee bubble again, and now I say it's OK. I think it does both parties good.

The staff room was also suggested as a suitable place for tears; for Ottily, this was where she found emotional support from her colleagues:

OTTILY: We all help and support each other when these things happen. You can have a little cry in the coffee room.

The emotional sustenance suggested by Ottily was also mentioned by Florrie in the form of refreshment, but this was more in the context of providing a route by which she could remove herself from the presence of the grieving mother:

FLORRIE: I think it's OK [to cry] . . . although she should not cry to the point of breaking down, maybe go out of the room, may be have a cup of tea in between, maybe go out and do other jobs.

Kerrie's attempts to remove herself from the grieving parents' presence appear to have actually served to open up the communication between her and the parents:

KERRIE: You can't burst into tears and you just have to . . . as I say sometimes they come outside the door and there you are having a wee cry to yourself and then you all go back in . . . y'know.

I have suggested that the sluice may be the appropriate place for crying in view of its function in disposing of waste. The midwives lead me to believe that crying is a more constructive activity, akin to finding sustenance. This may also be applied to the comments made by Zy, whose use of the changing room for crying helped to prepare her for a more open relationship with the parents. This more constructive interpretation of crying may also be found in the account of a poorly supported student nurse caring for a dying child (Anon, 1993), who found herself in tears in the ward kitchen, the place for preparing nourishment.

Control

The literature and quotations mentioned already show that some degree of ambivalence towards crying openly still exists among nurses and midwives. Although generally accepting of crying with a grieving mother, those mid-wives who were my informants invariably expressed some concern about whether they would be able to limit or control their crying. It may be that these midwives' underlying concerns about the acceptability of their crying, learned through nursing and midwifery training and years of practice, manifested themselves in the need to control this quintessentially uncontrollable act:

HILARY: I've been near to tears a couple of times . . . but you can't get too involved, you have got to have a cut-off point or else you wouldn't be able to handle it.

This cut-off point is a crucially important and recurring theme in midwives' accounts of the extent to which they allow themselves to cry. Effie mentions the self-awareness which is necessary if this self-imposed cut-off point is to operate:

EFFIE: I think it is fair enough for you to be grieving along with her as long as you are in control of the situation. . . . I think it may be quite a good thing for [the mother] that someone is there sharing the grief, so long as they are aware of what they are doing themselves. I think there is a situation where you can be upset along with someone but still remain professional.

As midwives we identify our own cut-off points, beyond which we fear being unable to function. The midwives spelt out the importance of identifying this point in terms of fearing going too far:

IRENE: I have cried many times. I don't totally break down, you really must keep control of the situation, but I would certainly shed a tear or two.

KAY: It's a very sad experience. And you should show them that you actually care and that it's not something that you do seven days of the week . . . I think there's crying and crying, and there's a few tears and having the screaming abdabs, and you're no use to anybody if you're like that.

ANNIE: I must admit I am quite an emotional person myself and obviously you don't want to get hysterical or anything like that. I'll be quite honest – I can't help myself shedding a few tears. You just have to make it very quiet and discreet and not . . . You don't want them having to feel sorry for you, which would obviously be totally inappropriate . . .

These comments by Kay and Annie show that their cut-off point has been fixed to prevent their crying causing their presence to be either unhelpful or counterproductive. The point identified by Annie was widely accepted among the midwives as the cut-off point, that is, when the parents need to support the midwife. Another criterion which the midwives use to help them to identify their own cut-off points was their ability to function effectively. This may be similar to the 'professionalism' already discussed, but some explained this concept in more helpful terms:

OTTILY: You can always cry with the couple. I think that the important thing is for you to be strong in order to be able to help them.

LEONIE: Sometimes it can be very draining on yourself emotionally, but the point at which you become no help to her is the point where it completely overtakes you. When you can't come into the room without getting terribly upset and being so upset, probably upsetting them further. We're in danger of that if we are not recognising that that is possible.

This point emphasises our need for the self-awareness mentioned already by Effie. Leonie built on her ideas about self-awareness by describing her impression of midwives' need for and awareness of clearly defined personal limits:

LEONIE: I think there has to be [limits], we have to know where they are, and maybe if we are getting to that stage or feel it's getting too much then we have to stop short because then we stop being any help. We stop being the pillar of support that the mother so desperately needs.

KAY: The last thing the mother needs is to be comforting somebody who is supposed to be helping her. But I don't think that a moist eye or a tear running down my cheek is going to do her any harm. Obviously if you feel that it's upsetting her then that is the time to withdraw, and just leave them on their own and get yourself together.

The midwife having to withdraw from the caring situation is something we have to consider if her ability to provide care is likely to be compromised by her emotional reaction to the mother's loss.

LEONIE: Maybe she can take time out . . . if there's two midwives then it's easier . . . the midwife then needs to go and talk it over with one of her fellow colleagues, get out her emotions about it . . . she can't bottle it up herself or I think she'd probably go off feeling very depressed and maybe not handle the next one quite so well . . .

The possibility of the midwife's emotional response causing her to withdraw from a grieving situation obviously has serious management and staffing implications, as well as the personal aspects already mentioned. Emotional factors are one of the areas which midwives need to take into account when the team leader is planning their work at the beginning of a shift:

LEONIE: If she feels that when the staff are allocated that this is a situation which at this particular time that she feels she couldn't quite handle, she could say 'I prefer not to look after this lady because I don't feel that I might be as supportive as somebody else might be given different circumstances.' This would apply if she was feeling more susceptible for some reason, there may be some background upset in her own life, where if there might have been a death of any member in the family then she's less likely . . . maybe she will understand but be less likely to be emotionally supportive, and more likely to feel the greater emotion herself, I don't know. She may be less able to give because she's still handling this experience, a similar experience herself and maybe hasn't come to terms with it enough in order to help this particular couple.

The need for the midwife to be in control of her crying emerged strongly, as did the anxiety that crying might impair the midwife's functioning. The midwives were able to differentiate very clearly the degree of crying which they regarded as permissible. They knew that red eyes or a quiet tear are quite in order, but any noisy or obvious displays of emotion would be counterproductive. Unfortunately, these extremes are both covered by the term 'crying'. Wagner and colleagues (1997) did not make this crucial distinction in their quantitative research, which means that the reader, and perhaps the respondents, experiences some uncertainty about the precise meaning of the term 'crying'.

The midwife's need to assume control over her behaviour may appear to contrast sharply with the midwife's wish to behave in a spontaneous or natural way when sharing the woman's grief. I suggest that this contrast is not real, as we need certain boundaries within which to operate if we are to allow ourselves to behave in a natural and human way.

Inability to cry

I have already touched on some of the management implications of the midwife sharing the mother's grief. These factors apply mainly in the labour ward setting, where one midwife would be caring for one grieving mother or couple. This emphasis is not inappropriate in view of the fact that, because of the likelihood of early transfer home, the labour ward is where a grieving mother spends most of her hospital stay.

In the postnatal ward the demands on the midwife's time are likely to be different, in that she may be caring less intensively, but for a larger number of mothers. If one of those mothers is grieving the loss of her baby, the midwife may encounter difficulties with the constant adjustment and readjustment between mothers in differing emotional states:

CARRIE: You have got to deal with this one woman, often due to staff allocations and the busyness of the ward, not only are you looking after this one grieving mother, partner, siblings, what have you, you've got to be next door with somebody who has had a nice bouncing baby and be happy for that person. It can be quite difficult sometimes to really have a chance to – or feel that you can – really express your feelings. A lot of the time it is so sad. All you want to do is to start crying for the woman and then you have to come out of the door and start coping with the rest of the ward and be seen to be in command. . . . It can be difficult.

This is clearly not just a short-term problem involving the midwife making adjustments between very different situations in which mothers' needs vary hugely. The longer-term implications for midwives of being prevented from expressing our feelings during the on-duty period need attention. This scenario places an intolerable strain on our informal support network, which may have lasting effects on us and those to whom we are close.

The inability to cry in a midwife working in a busy postnatal ward is similar to the account of the difficulties encountered by a junior house officer (Martin, 2000). Drawing on her experience of her father's death, she pleads for a more human and humane medical stereotype. Martin describes her 'horrendous hours, storing up the pain [of her grief] until it erupts in a flood of exhausted irritability when I come off duty'. In this description we see some aspects in common with the scenario of Carrie, mentioned above. Martin clearly spells out the adverse effects of her on-duty stress on her off-duty support network, which may be assumed to apply also to those close to the midwife.

Martin's search for insights into medical practitioners' difficulties may be illuminated by a philosophical paper by Adshead and Dickenson (1993). These writers probe the reasons for the 'contrasting approaches' taken by 'doctors and nurses' in the care of people who are dying. Whereas Martin refers to the medical practice of using science as a shield from reality, presumably another example of the defence mechanisms already mentioned, Adshead and Dickenson discuss medical reliance on the positivistic model, involving denying values and beliefs a place in science. These writers commend the more broadly based system of nursing education and the more heterogeneous population from which nursing students are likely to be drawn, implying a breadth of experience denied to their medical colleagues.

In her paper Martin regrets the 'outmoded macho image of invulnerability' still prevalent among her peers. Likewise, Adshead and Dickenson (1993) identify a 'cult of macho toughness' imbued during medical training, which is particularly stringent for female students. This issue becomes most poignant at the point where Martin, regretting her inability by virtue of her medical background to grieve openly, observes 'were I a nurse, a few tears would be permissable'. Adshead and Dickenson interpret Martin's observation in terms of the broad gender differences between nurses and medical practitioners, the tendency to tears being more stereotypically female in Western societies, allowing nurses to cry. It may be appropriate to question whether female nurses and midwives have assimilated the more masculine attitudes of our medical colleagues to this behaviour, in the same way as we may have assimilated other medical concepts.

The epidemiological data collected in Sweden by Rådestad and her colleagues (1996a) lend a quite objective view to this discussion. These data show the women's general satisfaction with the care which was provided for her and her stillborn baby at the time of the birth. They show, though, that, in spite of this general satisfaction, there was always a proportion of women who criticised the care which had been provided. Thus 9 per cent (29/310) of the mothers considered that the support given by medical staff in seeing and holding the dead baby was 'not at all' adequate. More disconcertingly, 32 per cent (100/309) wished that the medical staff had been more active in encouraging contact with the dead baby. Unsurprisingly, these researchers found that most of the women experienced emotional support from the baby's father. A slightly smaller proportion (65 per cent: 204/314) was supported by the midwife, whereas only 22 per cent (69/314) felt that any support was provided by the medical staff.

It is necessary to question whether the permissibility of tears observed by Martin might relate to the power relationship between the client and the carer. If this applies, a more equal or balanced relationship would reduce perceptions of vulnerability to allow openness in sharing grief. The data from my study indicate midwives' perceptions of partnership with those for whom they care, with the only exception being a few nagging doubts about being professional.

Summary

In this chapter I have discussed only our outward signs of grief. I have attempted neither to probe the feelings underlying these outward manifestations nor to describe the stress engendered among midwives and other staff caring for grieving mothers (see Chapter 10). A research project by Begley (2003) seeks to address the underlying emotions and their expression, albeit in student midwives.

In this chapter I have been able to make comparisons with the 'Projektgruppe Weinen' (Wagner *et al.*, 1997; Barth *et al.*, 2004). Unlike the midwives I interviewed, these researchers seem to regard crying as a problem. The midwives tended not to see it like that; to the midwives crying was perceived more as another mode of communication, being comparable with the other varieties of body language in their extensive repertoires. This, in turn, may reflect the uniformly female sample of midwives. Wagner and colleagues also distinguished their work by linking crying with distress and the need for support to the extent of seeking counselling. This is not the midwives' perception of what was, to them, a much more humdrum activity.

I have focused on the way in which crying helps staff members and the extent to which we consider that our tears facilitate the progress of the mother's grief. There has been little attention given to the physiological benefits of tears to the person who is crying (Dean, 1997). It appears from the data I have presented that, generally, midwives feel that increasing openness in sharing feelings about the loss of a baby is beneficial. We should treat this statement cautiously, though. This is because of, for example, the seriously limited research-based English-language literature on this uniquely sensitive topic.

12 Self-help support groups

I became aware, during my research on mothers who do not have their babies with them (Mander, 1995b), of the importance midwives attach to self-help groups' contribution to the care of a grieving mother. The benefits have been demonstrated in the general self-help literature. Research by, among others, Kaunonen and colleagues (1999), Parkes (1980) and Raphael (1984), focusing on the loss of a spouse, has shown the benefits of a secure social support network, including self-help groups. There has been little research, however, on support for grieving parents (Chambers and Chan, 2004).

In this chapter I focus on perinatal self-help support groups. To do this, I briefly consider what self-help involves; then, in order to apply this material to perinatal bereavement, I use as a framework the observations which midwives made during my study. Next, the role of health care providers and hospital-based self-help support groups is considered. The contribution of internet support is then explored. Finally, I address outstanding issues and attempt to probe the benefits of self-help, by drawing on the scant evaluative research literature. Inevitably, because of the dearth of specific material, I am compelled to draw on the literature relating to self-help more generally than perinatal loss.

I use the term 'self-help' to differentiate this support from that offered by health care providers, which is the primary focus of this book. The interface between the support which health care providers offer and that provided by others deserves attention because it is here that our care of the grieving mother may be found wanting.

Lay support systems include a more informal sector, the family and friends, which is highly individual, as well as the less informal sector on which I focus here. This latter more organised system of lay support or self-help comprises groups which are established to help the members deal or cope with a common problem, in this context perinatal grief. It is widely accepted that it is the 'helper-therapy principle' which operates to ensure the success of self-help; this means that people who help others are likely to experience benefits for themselves. Self-help has been usefully defined in terms of five crucial features:

- members have a common difficulty in their life
- the group is run by the members without external support
- the members meet for mutual benefit
- there is an element of formality in the organisation of the group
- subscriptions or contributions may be paid, but no fees are involved.

(Wilson, 1995: 4)

This phenomenon has also been termed 'mutual aid' as well as 'lay support', but 'self-help' is the currently preferred term (Adamsen and Rasmussen, 2001). A well-known and longstanding example is Alcoholics Anonymous (White, 2004). The breadth and variation of interpretation of 'self-help' becomes apparent in the work of Simonds (2002) on maternity care. She quotes a variety of experts, ranging from obstetricians, such as DeLee, to birth activists, such as Sheila Kitzinger.

Historical background

While attempting to disentangle the twin concepts of self-care and self-help, Kickbusch (1989) outlines the development of self-help. Our growing interest in self-help resulted from the growth of medical sociology in the 1950s and 1960s which, in turn, was a response to increasing medical power. At a more personal level, the balance of power in the traditional 'patient–physician' relationship began to be questioned in the work of writers such as Illich (1976). The growth of self-help was fuelled by social movements, such as the women's movement, which exposed concerns about the 'medicalisation' of healthy processes, such as childbearing.

Kickbusch asserts that self-help became more firmly established with the consumerist ethos of the 1970s. During this decade mutual learning and support was the philosophy which was preferred in comparison to more medical approaches. Our growing realisation that each of us is the expert when it comes to our own functioning carried connotations of self-control and empowerment, causing the power balance in health care interactions to change. The more equal inputs carry an aura of assertiveness, which may be seen by some as a threat to the traditional, one-sided arrangement of professional dominance in the medical model. Kickbusch compares the concurrent moves from a disease to a health orientation and from a medical to a self-help approach. These upheavals were recognised in the publication of a community health care programme (WHO, 1983). Since this seal of approval from WHO, self-help has assumed even greater significance in the UK. Adams (1996), using a social work perspective, demonstrates how self-help has contributed to patients and clients assuming control over their circumstances, that is, their empowerment. Thus, it is clear that the self-help movement has, since its inception, been imbued with obvious political overtones (Burns and Taylor, 1998).

The activities of self-help groups are susceptible to misunderstanding and unrealistic expectations, which is a major reason for the demise of some potentially effective groups. Knowledge of the basic functions of a self-help group would help ensure a common purpose; these include reduction of isolation, facilitating problem-solving, sharing coping skills, identifying other sources of help, improving confidence, empowering people to improve their own lives, giving emotional support, providing alternatives to medication, organising social contacts, undertaking pressure group activities and public consciousness-raising.

Self-help in the context of perinatal grief

When asked about the support available for the grieving mother, the midwives I interviewed (Mander, 1995b) mentioned professionals, family and various forms of self-help. Here I relate the midwives' comments to the literature on self-help in both general situations and in the context of perinatal grief.

Benefiting

The midwives were generally confident that the grieving mother would benefit from contact with a mother who had experienced a similar loss and also through being involved with a support group:

RM: What would you say is the aim of midwives' care for this mother?

QUEENY: You can tell them about SANDS. I think the contact with other bereaved mothers is helpful.

IRENE: In terms of the long-term care of this mother we are able to put her in touch with societies formed by mothers who have experienced a similar problem. There are support groups that would be able to help her or it may be possible to put her into contact directly with a mother I know who has been through a similar experience. I think that they are helpful to this mother.

LUCY: I think there is a lot of other methods of support that we have to give her as well. Sometimes that can be just sitting talking to her, other times it can take the form of actual support groups that are available for women in these circumstances. We would give them advice, or there are sisters working in the paediatric department – if her baby has been in the paediatric department – then they would be able to deal with all the different support groups that may be applicable to that person.

Making contact

Establishing contact with others in a similar situation is the first step in the 'self-help process' (Adams, 1990). He describes joining an established group or, alternatively, identifying with a like-minded person the need to initiate a new group. Either way, an essential precursor is the realisation that a problem exists and that, with the help of others, it may be manageable.

Passing on information to a grieving mother about local groups was clearly seen as part of midwifery care:

IZZY: I have, though, referred people to SANDS organisation. We have their telephone number in the ward. And I give her the telephone number before she goes.

BETTY: I think it is useful to put the bereaved mother in touch with a contact person [for a support group] before she is discharged.

Apart from comments such as these, little is written about how the grieving mother learns of the existence and potential benefits of self-help support groups.

Being 'caught in a trap' is how a grieving mother may feel when she is ready and able to talk about her grief. The reason for her feeling cornered is that the midwife will have stopped visiting and her partner will have returned to work. In this situation a support group plays an important role:

GAY: She felt she could've had somebody else to talk to. And she said that by the time she was ready to talk about it, there was nobody coming in to see her, y'know. And that was hard for her. Yeah, a self-help group probably would help, yes. And then it's trying to encourage a person to actually go and phone. They think they will probably cause a nuisance. Yeah, I think they would help.

Feelings of being trapped may be aggravated by the grieving mother's difficulty in preparing herself physically and psychologically to make the first move.

Making an out-of-the-blue approach to begin a relationship is especially daunting when a mother's grief makes her isolated and vulnerable. The woman is likely to hesitate and procrastinate before making that initial contact. Penson (1990) details the 'emotional energy' necessary for a bereaved woman to make this first move and how she may 'put off telephoning for several days'. It may be possible to help ease this first painful and tentative step:

AMY: Another thing that you can do is guide them towards SANDS, and explain to them what it is and that if they need help they can get in touch with them or we can get in touch with them for them. Y'know . . . like breaking the ice.

Thus, some midwives tried to make that difficult first move. It is impossible to judge whether her helpfulness was successful or whether the mother's anxiety was simply transferred to another stage further along in the joining process.

Caution was expressed by some midwives, although almost invariably they spoke positively about self-help support groups. The cautious midwives felt that some mothers would not be helped by these groups, either because of the nature of the group or the characteristics of the mother herself:

SHIRLEY: They can be very helpful. I think an awful lot depends on how well she has been counselled and how much help she needs. Some people do need the extra help and the support of outsiders. Some people would resent outsiders knowing what they would term 'their business'. They would term it 'interference'. You've got to take it very carefully. You've got to decide – I have given out these addresses of self-help groups to mothers, but there are other odd mothers I have never approached with it because I know they wouldn't take to it.

Shirley was unable to explain the characteristics in a mother that would make her decide not to impart this information. A very experienced midwife, having worked with mothers and babies for over thirty years, Shirley drew on empathy, intuition and gut feeling for many of her care decisions, including this one.

Health care providers clearly have some input into how grieving mothers learn about support groups, although feelings about who would want to join such a group influence whether information is given.

Joining and not joining

The variation in the nature and organisation of self-help groups means that the concept of formal membership may not always be relevant, but becoming part of the group is not even possible until the person has at least gone to a meeting. Like Shirley, mentioned above, some midwives emphasised the voluntary nature of support groups and the possibility that some mothers would not be keen to become involved:

DOROTHY: They've got support groups for them. Some of them like to have phone numbers and some of them aren't the least bit interested. They've got them if they need it.
GINNIE: I think it is a voluntary thing for the patient and her partner. If they want to contact SANDS they can.
TRUDY: I think they have a role to play . . . I think it is the ultimate role often . . . I think it has a role and I think if the individual is wanting to go, that's great.

A common criticism of self-help is highlighted by both Adams (1990) and Layne (1999), which may explain the reluctance of some individuals to join groups. From his UK standpoint, Adams relates modern self-help to the bourgeois, paternalistic, charitable movements of the Victorian era and links the two phenomena by socio-economic class, claiming that self-help 'has often reflected the values of middle-class society'. Adams's contention contrasts with the view that self-help originated with the trade unions (Miller and Webb, 1988) and, hence, is a working-class phenomenon. Layne's participant observation research in the USA supports Adams's view, having found that there the 'membership is predominantly white and middle class' (1999: 177).

It is necessary to conclude that the reasons for people not joining support groups may relate, first, to the lack of a suitable group or ignorance of its existence. Second, a person may decide not to join, either because they have the help they need, or because they fear being unwelcome or out of place.

Her misgivings at the prospect of joining a support group are recounted by a widow who was a psychotherapist (Rose, 1990). Categorising herself as an elitist non-joiner, she contemplates the value of support to groups of people to which she definitely does not belong, such as 'alcoholics and lost souls'. Her professional self increased the distance by reminding her that she was 'the therapist, not the patient'. Rose describes her fear of loss of uniqueness which group membership would bring, in that she was unprepared to recognise that others may have a not identical but similar experience. She eventually realised that her defences had protected her well in the early stages of her grief, but were in danger of isolating her and aggravating her sorrow. Rose had particular difficulty with the notion that she needed the help of a group, but eventually resolved her aversion.

Penson (1990) suggests that a bereaved person may not wish to attend or join due to fear of a 'morbid' atmosphere, when the only common factor is the death of someone close. Alternatively, knowing that self-disclosure is a feature of support groups, some people may feel unready to discuss their experience. As a way of dealing with these fears, a range of non-threatening ice-breaking techniques may be used to help new members to 'open up'. There are also the crucially important group activities which are less grief-related, in order to increase the group's cohesion and fun pursuits, to counter fears of a morbid atmosphere (Klass, 1997).

A successful support group needs to have certain characteristics which make people comfortable attending it. These include allowing each of the members both space and opportunities for contact. Self-esteem and confidence-building are fundamental to the ultimate achievement of independence for each group member. These characteristics are as relevant to a perinatal support group as to any other.

Being in a crisis

YOLANDY: ... all of a sudden they're faced with a situation they can't cope with and it's something they've got to get used to, and it's easier if they can talk to somebody else who has been through the same situation. Reassuring for them as well, because I think a lot of the ladies get very frightened and the reactions they're having to the situation that they find themselves in. They're going through the grieving process. A lot of these young girls have never known bereavement in a family situation.

Although she did not mention the word, Yolandy's account of the grieving mother's feelings brings to mind both the lay and the more psychologically oriented concept of a crisis. The suddenness of the event is combined with the unexpected inability to cope with it, reminiscent of Caplan's definition: 'A crisis is provoked when a person faces an obstacle to important life goals that is, for a time, insurmountable through customary methods of problem-solving' (1961). Mutual aid, self-help and support groups are recognised as having a role in crisis situations. Another of these roles, identification of the person's own strengths, has much in common with the self-help ethos, as does the final outcome – independent functioning.

A more mundane view of crisis and the self-help response may be associated with the increasingly finite resources of the formal care sector. For this reason, help may be absent when the person most needs it; alternatively, an urgent appointment or referral may be impossible. This scenario contrasts with the availability of self-help contacts, whose experience of similar problems means that help is accessible immediately and freely. Many groups take the provision of direct help a stage further by encouraging the perception of being supported and by offering help before it has been sought.

Self-help and the health care system

The direct help offered by self-care groups, in contrast with the limited resources of the health care system, provides us with an example of how self-help and formal health care interact.

The overlap between self-help and formal health care

The overlap between support groups' help and formal care provision emerged in the midwives' comments. They were aware of the lack of resources, and considered that support groups would be able to fill the gap. To this extent they regarded the self-help groups as complementary to the formal services:

GINNIE: I think you have to be very understanding . . . and you have to accept the fact that, should they require more counselling than you can actually give them, you must be ready to hand over care of these patients to SANDS or such a group of people.

Likewise, the relative inadequacy of statutory provision was recognised by 'officials', who envied the lack of bureaucracy and the immediacy of response in self-help groups (Richardson and Goodman, 1983). Despite this, these researchers concluded that the role of self-help is to supplement formal care, as the consumers in their sample utilised professional help, by consulting 'various medical experts, social workers and advice officers'. They used self-help groups for mutual support or when needing the understanding of someone who had personal experience of a situation, leading to the authors' assertion that self-help's unique strength lies in its reciprocity:

WENDY: There are other people there you can talk to who've been through the same experience. They really understand. I've heard on one occasion the comment that [the staff] 'were so nice and tried to be so understanding, but they really don't know how I feel' and I think that having places like SANDS they are talking to people who really do know what they are feeling and who have been through it themselves; that's bound to help . . .

The supplementary nature of self-help also emerged:

TRUDY: I think there is an awful lot more that could be done. I don't think we should just say which is the . . . 'Here's the baby's registration, funeral bits and here is the self-help organisations . . .' Not that it does in reality actually happen like that, but I still think . . . there's more . . .

It is clear from the midwives that they regard self-help as an important adjunct to their care, to the extent that it provides more extensive and longer-term care than they are able to offer, in fact the partnership which is earnestly sought in the social work field. It is possible, however, for the implications of this 'partnership' to be interpreted less benignly, in that the spectre of manipulation arises. Self-help may be used as a political football to either justify cutbacks in health and social services or to encourage individual self-sufficiency and prosperity (Adams, 1990).

Lack of groups

Examining the data and the literature on support groups brings me to consider resources, as raised by Betty in response to my open question:

RM: What changes do you think are needed in the care of this mother?
BETTY: More bereavement support groups would be helpful.

Ginnie also observed the shortage of this form of care and was able to deduce both the immediate and underlying reasons:

GINNIE: . . . unfortunately they don't seem to have enough . . . of them. We have a list of contacts but obviously if these ladies have other family they stop working for SANDS because of their own reasons, but I think it is like everything else – they are really underfunded.

Limited provision is similarly observed and regretted by Leon (1990), who considers that a dearth of counselling services exists in all areas of bereavement support, despite its value in some areas having been well established by research.

Reciprocal helping

I have already mentioned that mutual support based on common experience, or reciprocity, is the unique strength of self-help; but whether someone experiencing difficulty is best placed to support others in the same situation is questionable. It may be that a person struggling to manage her own life may lack the emotional energy to support another. This conundrum may be solved by the concept of 'serial reciprocity' which is fundamental to self-help. This involves those, in whom a longer time has elapsed from their experience, being better able to support those who are newly afflicted. Thus, the people who attend group meetings may initially do so because they hope to receive support, information, direct help or social contacts. As they become more confident within the group and their problem resolves, they find themselves able to give more. This may be in the form of advice and support to relatively new members or as a commitment to organising the group.

A midwife explained this concept:

IRENE: . . . people's roles may be reversed; the bereaved couple having been helped may better find that they are able to help others in a similar situation. The group may not be of any help immediately after the birth, but she may be the sort of woman who wants to grieve alone and then maybe contact such a group later when she is ready to. She may find that she is better able to give support at that stage to other women who have lost their babies, rather than being the one who accepts others' support.

Irene distinguishes women who benefit once or twice from belonging to a group. The twice-benefiting woman is supported initially and later gains satisfaction from supporting others; whereas another woman may benefit only once, on the later occasion. Whereas Irene presents serial reciprocity as a dichotomy, it may be viewed as a continuum comparable with grieving. At one end of the continuum the mother is immersed in her grief and able only to accept support, but as her grieving progresses she needs less support and is able to give more. She eventually reaches the other end of the continuum when her grief is more integrated into her life and her support needs have diminished. At this point she has a wealth of experience of both grieving and being supported, enabling her to help others. The research project by Klass (1997), on the place of The Compassionate Friends (TCF) in the progress of grief, shows how the parents' role changes with time until they begin to forget some aspects of the group's activities. This forgetfulness, about the group rather than the dead child, indicates to them that they are ready to move away from the group. Klass explains this phenomenon in terms of the parents' relationship with their dead child becoming more secure, while their link with TCF weakens.

Hospital-based support groups

I have been emphasising the mutuality of support through self-help, in that shared experience underpins empathy. The extent to which professional carers who have not shared this experience are able to facilitate group support now deserves attention. The midwives I interviewed did not claim that hospital-based support groups were self-help groups, but their existence leads us to think about the input of the formal carers:

DEIDRE: Special Care has got parents' support groups and things. They don't have a counsellor but they do have groups.

HILARY: There is a society in this unit for parents who have been bereaved. It is run by two of the sisters and each bereaved mother is sent a personal invitation to ask her to come along to the group which meets monthly in the hospital.

A bereavement group was set up in a maternity unit by midwifery staff and named the 'Care and Support Circle' (Priest, 2000: 185). The role of the carers in initiating the group and inviting bereaved parents is described, as well as some of the pitfalls which lie in wait for the well-meaning. The increasing involvement of the midwifery staff appears to be welcomed by the bereaved parents at the 'services' which are being held annually. The pervasive Christian orientation of these services has been strengthened, though, in spite of adverse comments by some bereaved parents. This leads to concerns about whether some grieving parents may effectively be being excluded from the benefits of these midwives' efforts. Adamsen and Rasmussen (2001) suggest that professional involvement in such groups may serve to feed back views about care generally in order to improve services.

The implications for professionals in self-help groups should not be underestimated. This is mainly because the entire ethos of self-help is founded on the primacy of experiential, that is, non-expert, knowledge (Adamsen and Rasmussen, 2001).

Adams (1996), like Kickbusch (1989), emphasises that the assumption of control by the client group carries the inevitable implication that control must be relinquished by another group. Obviously, those relinquishing power are the professional carers; this change in the balance of power may not only be threatening to professionals, but be likely to 'complicate' or damage the relationship between the consumer, that is the client or patient, and her formal carer. That self-help usually evolves to satisfy needs left unmet by deficiencies or gaps in formal provision does little to alleviate professionals' feelings of threat.

These anxieties or uncertainties about the hazards and benefits of self-help may be resolved by some professionals by their focus on the marginality of self-help. Thus, they regard it as just a fringe activity or possibly as a harmless diversion. Such professionals are likely to decide that it can usually be safely ignored. Professionals' difficulty in understanding the concept of self-help is likely to be aggravated by the short-term and friable nature of some groups, the diversity of the problems addressed and the multiplicity of members' expectations. The inability to 'pigeon-hole' self-help into traditional health care models clearly does not facilitate outsiders' understanding.

Such difficulties tend to be discounted by Adamsen and Rasmussen (2001) who envisage self-help as a growth area ripe for professional input, if not control. These researchers report their findings as showing that 84 per cent of self-help participants 'request professional involvement' (2001: 912). The extent of this involvement, they admit, varies from being part of the group to a loose affiliation on a consultancy basis. These writers go on to quote other authorities who emphasise that the non-professional stance of self-help is no longer feasible. Thus, it appears that attempts are being made to professionalise self-help, which is a total anathema to its basic principles and origins. Clearly such a development would endanger the mutuality of the group and totally alter the form of interaction within the group. Were Adamsen and Rasmussen's recommendations to be implemented, such group activity would become little more than an adjunct to the already over-medicalised orthodox health care system.

The development of one self-help bereavement support group by a professional is detailed by the nurse involved (Penson, 1990). She explains how unique nursing skills may be used to found and establish the group, including finding a suitable venue, identifying potential members and creating a warm and encouraging atmosphere. Penson summarises the nurse's function as being to facilitate contact, by bringing together those who need help and those who can offer it. Contrary to the assertions above, she then goes on to emphasise the need for the nurse to withdraw from the group, allowing it to continue to evolve as determined by the members. The professional may continue to be available to act as a trouble-shooter in the event of problems, but distance appears to be vital.

Adopting an unashamedly political orientation, Adams (1990) probes the difficulties which professionals are likely to encounter when, because of limited resources, the inevitable increase in self-help requires them to relinquish power to newly empowered consumers. Such a realignment may give rise to feelings of threat among some professionals. Their difficulty may be due to the traditional professional view of self-help as 'at best wasteful of resources and at worst downright counterproductive'.

Although self-help is viewed positively by those I interviewed, there is an element of caution, if not anxiety, underlying professional responses to it. This applies in spite of benefits which accrue for carers from groups' activities.

A feature of self-help groups which was of importance to the midwives I interviewed but which does not appear in the general self-help literature relates to **the assistance which they provide for carers**. This may be in the form of information, which operates at two levels. The first level is the provision of feedback on the care provided for the grieving mother:

ZY: I've being thinking about going along . . . to find out what the women felt themselves about what we all did for them . . . how we helped or what we can still do to help.

BESSIE: The only thing . . . was a reading list I got. I'm not sure where it came from. I think it might have been SANDS . . . the talk by the people from SANDS also helped. I was able to get a lot of feedback about my care of these women through SANDS.

The need for us to learn of mothers' views to inform care, otherwise only available by research, is crucial. The second level at which self-help groups assist midwives is in their information and literature and through formal and informal face-to-face contacts. Although the printed material is designed to be distributed to grieving mothers, it is not unreasonable that the carer should read the material first, if only to ensure that it is acceptable:

GINNIE: I read the SANDS stuff that they have. It's very good literature that they hand out to the patients about various . . . it's a question and answer type thing and it's showing you questions that partners are asking and other people have asked and I've found that very helpful.

The gifts of equipment and other resources which self-help groups donate to maternity units serve to influence practice, as well as supporting the staff:

ZY: I think [groups] probably will be helpful. I know the lady, the contact that we have, that we got the Moses basket through. She's a very nice lady, and she's very helpful, even just for us to talk to. . . .

HATTIE: Oh, SANDS are good, very good. They have given us a book of remembrance which is very nice.

That health care providers need to rely on self-help groups for such basic items of equipment may be a reflection on the priorities of the UK health care system.

Internet self-help support groups

Unlike grief counselling more generally, the use of internet support in situations of perinatal loss is relatively under-developed. A search using Google produced a large number of 'hits', whereas the insertion of 'perinatal' into the search term reduced the number of hits drastically, and many of those were culturally inappropriate. The SANDS website, although using electronic communication, strongly encourages those seeking support to use the telephone helpline (SANDS, 2004).

A number of issues relating to internet support groups were encountered in an ethnographic research on older people (Eley, 2003). Eley collected data from both virtual (on-line) and actual (off-line) support groups. Additionally, she undertook electronic and face-to-face interviews respectively. She found that her informants were very comfortable with internet support, particularly in view of the 'ordinariness of the talk', being with 'like-minded people', talking to 'people who really understand' and being in a 'safe place to talk'. The safety issue, although identified by both sets of informants, had different meanings for each set. For the actual group, safety was found in the reputation of the organisation which had facilitated the establishment of the group. On the other hand, for the virtual group members, safety lay in their ability to control their degree or extent of personal disclosure. This meant that they valued being able to retain their anonymity, or dispense with it for some messages, and also the ability to 'lurk' unheard and unobserved.

A literature review of research on health-related computer-mediated support groups identified issues which may be relevant to those concerned with perinatal loss (Wright and Bell, 2003). In the matter of on-line support, these researchers note the importance of a sense of community within the group. They question how a virtual group is able to create such a feeling and whether it is associated with better, that is, healthier, outcomes. A further, not unrelated, question emerges in these researchers' consideration of the on-line group member's interaction with her actual support network. The implication is that her actual support system, such as her family, may be offering her support which is very different from her on-line supporters, with the potential for conflict and serious harm to her grieving process. As mentioned below, evaluation of their effects should be a priority for this form of self-help support group, particularly in view of the mushrooming of these internet sites. Such evaluation has been shown, however, to be an ethical minefield (Eysenbach and Till, 2001).

Issues

As mentioned already, some midwives were cautious about recommending a grieving mother to attend a self-help group because the mother might not fit in with the group and might be hurt by the experience.

The activities of the group possibly being unhelpful also caused concern to some midwives:

RUBY: There is a . . . organisation called SANDS. I think they are very good. I think they do a lot of good. But some of them maybe go a little over the top, and get taken over by the kinds of woman who focus their minds too much on their grief.

Ruby's caution was based on her own observation, but Polly had been a midwife for over thirty years and drew on her own experience of having a stillborn baby to support her suggestion that a self-help group may be responsible for actually perpetuating the mother's grief:

POLLY: I had a stillbirth myself . . . when I came here there was a group from SANDS and they came down. They were talking, there was a group talking to the midwives about what their group did. I found it very harrowing. Even after all those years, I found that harrowing because I thought to myself 'I wouldn't have liked that.' As I say, I thought to myself I wouldn't have liked it if that had been offered to me. Of course in those days there was no such things as support groups. But I wouldn't have liked it. I felt that it wasn't really healthy that they should be just making this a big thing in their life. What worries me is the effect on the mums. That's what worries me. Because I try to put myself . . . I try to remember what it was like, and I wouldn't have liked it. They spoke about how they felt and how this happened and that happened and I felt it was as if they were grabbing on to this instead of trying to get over it. That was just how I felt. I really thought it was a bit unhealthy. I found it off-putting, I really did.

The possibility that self-help groups may be counterproductive to the extent that they may serve to prevent the grieving woman from moving forward in her grief could be a real problem. More recent views of the benefits of not moving on (Walter, 1999; see Chapter 1) resonate powerfully with self-help principles. The process sometimes known as 'biography' involves the grieving person making space in their life for the one who is lost. This contrasts with the usual stage process of working to 'let go' of the person and the memories.

That self-help groups are organised by lay people may serve to increase their sensitivity to the needs of their members, but difficulties may arise which may appear insoluble to people with little experience of group functioning. Tensions within the group may result in power struggles which reduce its effectiveness. On the other hand, if professionals are involved they may be used and allow themselves to be used inappropriately excessively. Assuming that the group is successful in resolving the concerns of the members, it may not know how to end itself in a constructive way, that is, by passing on its knowledge to others who are at an earlier stage in the process.

An assumption which underpins self-help is the significance of mutuality of experience, in that a person who has been through devastating grief, such as the loss of a baby, is considered better able to help and support another person going through it. This perception emerges forcefully in a qualitative study from Finland (Laakso and Paunonen-Ilmonen, 2002), in which the mothers thought that their experience of losing a child could only be shared by someone with a similar experience. I venture to suggest, however, that the assumption that 'my grief is your grief' may deny the uniqueness of the other person's feelings and, perhaps, even trivialise them.

This assumption emerges in Howarth and Leaman's discussion of issues relating to self-help (2001), and they extend it to suggest that bereaved people may only be effectively supported by those who have suffered a similar loss. The danger in this assumption was brought home to me when my own father died and a well-meaning colleague wrote a condolence note telling me of her father's death two years earlier and how she knew what I was feeling. The differences between her background and mine were too vast for there to be any common ground, and her presumptuousness further confused my already muddled feelings. Such assumptions, however, feature prominently among bereavement self-help groups and may actually serve to divide the adherents to different forms of interventions (Howarth and Leaman, 2001). With these caveats in mind, I suggest that we recognise the assumption of commonality for what it is and handle it cautiously.

The place of the father is possibly clearer in the context of self-help support groups than in other aspects of childbearing. It may not be surprising that Layne (1999, 2003) in her fieldwork in New York and New Jersey found that the man's attendance is 'strongly encouraged' by some support groups. This fits the picture of the North American father being *required* to support his partner in the latter stages of childbearing (Mander, 2001c). This father's involvement extends to his contribution to certain organisations' newsletters. McCreight (2004) in Northern Ireland identified some common themes with Layne in her qualitative study of the impact of pregnancy loss on the male partner. These commonalities may have been associated with McCreight's sampling, which comprised the members of six different pregnancy loss self-help groups. While McCreight is appropriately cautious not to generalise her findings, she shows the way in which the male partner appears to be particularly comfortable in assuming a leadership role in the organisation of the self-help group. This role extends beyond the organisation of meetings and the newsletters mentioned by Layne, making plans for events such as memorial services. McCreight contrasts these men's instrumental role with the tendency for these men's grief to be 'belittled or at least discounted' (2004: 343). She goes on to recognise these men's potential to change practice in maternity units. At the same time McCreight, like Layne, acknowledges the difficulty which men encounter in attending pregnancy loss self-help groups without their female partner. This means that, effectively, the woman is acting as a gatekeeper to allow her partner to assume this crucially influential role. McCreight goes on to discuss the influence of the man on the group's activities. She found that half of the groups she observed were facilitated jointly by a couple. Bereaved men were prepared to accompany their partners to these groups and to contribute. They were acutely uncomfortable attending a group led by a woman, commenting that 'I felt like it was a sort of woman's group' (2004: 344).

Evaluation

It is clear that, with only a few words of caution, midwives are happy to inform grieving mothers of the existence and role of perinatal bereavement support groups. It is necessary to ask, though, to what extent midwives' confidence is justified. In the same way as any intervention should be evidence-based, we should recognise the need for evaluation of the contribution of these groups. Research into their functioning, however, is notable mainly by its flawed research design (Kato and Mann, 1999) and also by its scarcity.

A relatively acceptable example, though, is found in the work of Lieberman (1979) who, with his colleagues, studied seven different self-help groups, including The Compassionate Friends (TCF), a group for bereaved parents. Lieberman's data, though, focus on bereaved parents' reasons for joining TCF, rather than on the outcomes or benefits of their contribution.

A researcher who had earlier been associated with the work of Lieberman found that involvement with TCF served to protect the parents from the development of emotional problems (Videka-Sherman, 1982). She found that parents who had lost a child through death within the previous eighteen months and were more active in the group were less likely to be depressed one year after the death than a similar group who contributed less to the organisation of the group and the support of other members. In interpreting these findings we must beware of assuming causality, as those parents who experienced their loss less severely, and perhaps were less depressed, may have been better able to help the other group members.

A Finnish study focusing on the mother's social support after the death of a child collected some data which constitute a certain degree of evaluation of support groups (Laakso and Paunonen-Ilmonen, 2002). As mentioned by McCreight (2004) and Layne (1999, 2003), these researchers identified men's difficulty in attending a grief support group. The mothers, though, articulated quite extreme reactions to their group involvement. The group was either supportive or unhelpful to the extent of being anxiety provoking (2002: 181). Those with a negative response compared themselves unfavourably with more articulate group members.

The quantitative research by DiMarco and her colleagues (2001) sought to evaluate the effectiveness of a perinatal loss support group (see Chapter 3). As with so much grief research, the sample was less than ideal. Their use of the Hogan Grief Reaction Checklist indicated no significant difference between the supported and the unsupported groups. Four of the six variables, however, showed better results for the unsupported, including despair, personal growth, detachment and disorganisation. The researchers conclude that a coping scale might have been a preferable instrument.

Researching the parents' experience of grief with the support of a self-help group would be highly sensitive, but evaluation research has been completed in other, similarly sensitive, areas; examples include the work of

O'Connor and colleagues (2003). The dilemmas and pitfalls of such sensitive, grief-related research, such as attrition and low response rates, are well recognised.

It appears that midwives are recommending self-help, as a way of assisting grieving parents in adjusting to their loss, on the basis of flawed research which suggests that this intervention does not improve outcomes (Kato and Mann, 1999). Inadequate knowledge of the functioning and benefits of self-help, in this context, render the midwife vulnerable (Chalmers, 1993). It is, thus, imperative that we should undertake research into the effectiveness of this form of support, perhaps by seeking the views of those with good experiences of such a group and comparing their ideas with those whose experience was less satisfactory.

Summary

While the presence of self-help groups is much valued by midwives and appears to be beneficial, we must listen to the words of caution which come from a range of sources; these include the warning of Kalish (1985): 'This does not mean that participation in death-related self-help groups never leads to serious disturbance . . . such participation is extremely low risk and the potential rewards are substantial.'

13 Future childbearing

For reasons that I do not fully understand, the question of a future pregnancy invariably arises when health care providers consider perinatal loss. Although I never raised the topic, many of the midwives in my research project (Mander, 1995b) thought that it was important to tell me about the prospect of the grieving mother embarking on another pregnancy. Some midwives illustrated how much our ideas have changed by disparagingly quoting 'traditional' advice:

ANNIE: 'You can have another baby. You are young yet. It doesn't really matter.'

In quoting this comment, Annie was criticising the way it trivialises the mother's experience and denies the uniqueness of her lost baby (Côté-Arsenault and Dombeck, 2001). Such words were presumably intended originally to reassure the mother and to persuade her to think positively about the future, rather than dwell on the past. It may have, thus, been intended to 'cure', or at least curtail, the mother's grief. That this view still exists was impressed upon me by the relinquishing mothers I interviewed, many of whom were being or had been encouraged to consider the therapeutic value of another pregnancy. Ursula's son was eight weeks old when we spoke and her anger and sorrow were still painfully obvious. This led her family to try to help:

URSULA: Everybody round about keeps advising me to have another child to make me feel better. But I'm not going to have a child as a form of therapy.

In this chapter I address the obstacles facing the woman who decides to resume her childbearing career. They are addressed in the chronological order in which they may present.

Resuming sexual intercourse

Although the subsequent pregnancy has been the subject of much attention, the method of conception, sexual intercourse, has been largely neglected. The difficulty of re-establishing a loving, sexual relationship following perinatal death is apparent mainly from mothers' personal anecdotes.

It may be difficult for a couple to enjoy even the human contact which may be quite independent of love-making. Physical comfort and support may be too much to ask of someone who feels they have nothing left to give. Even gentle warmth and undemanding cuddles require a degree of relaxation which may be hard for a grieving parent.

Sexual intimacy following the death of a child has been shown to be problematical by Singg (2003). She suggests that, while physical comfort may be appreciated, sexual intercourse is unlikely to be resumed until the couple are planning another pregnancy.

Differing patterns and rates of grieving may compound this difficulty because one partner is unable to respond to the other's tentative advances. Similarly, each partner's feelings of 'being ready for it', in terms of either grieving or simply inclination, may not coincide, escalating a cycle of tension and avoidance. Their resumption of sexual intercourse is likely to be delayed, as for any new parents, by the mother's traumatised genital area, lack of vaginal lubrication and any perineal damage.

Hidden meanings exist in sexual intercourse for a couple who are grieving. An example is their memories of love-making, some months earlier, which began their baby's all-too-brief existence, recalling a more joyful and more carefree time. The pleasurable nature of love-making may, thus, be regarded as inappropriate. It is possible to understand the perilous vicious cycle moving from 'I don't feel like it' to 'How could we?' to 'How could you think of it?'

The physical act of intercourse may serve as a further reminder of the birth and the death, as two mothers recounted (Kohner and Henley, 1992): 'She was the last person inside me and I didn't want to wipe out any part of that sacred memory.' 'Every time we make love I relive the birth.'

For either partner, fear of beginning another pregnancy, which has the potential for further trauma, may deter them from seeking the comfort of love-making. Although many couples deeply regret their inability to give each other intimate, loving support when they most need it, some couples may actually be relieved that the anxiety which sex brings with it has been removed. For those couples who regret the loss of the pleasurable comfort which sexual intimacy brings, this may be regarded as a secondary loss which prevents an activity which might alleviate, albeit momentarily, the sorrow of bereavement.

A research project undertaken in the USA (Swanson *et al.*, 2003) attempted to describe the effect of one particular form of loss on the couple's relationship. These researchers used a series of postal surveys and quantitative analysis to assess the extent of the development of the couples' interpersonal and sexual relationships in the first year after miscarriage. The researchers found that, for both relationships, for about half of the respondents there was no change. The number who stated that the relationships had improved were in a small minority, whereas those whose relationships had deteriorated constituted about one-third of the respondents. On the basis of these findings the researchers recommend that the couple should be prepared to cope with these changes in their interpersonal relationship. It is necessary to bear in mind, though, that these researchers did not collect any data from any male partners, so the picture is entirely one-sided.

Desiring to begin another pregnancy

The wish to begin another pregnancy may be interpreted differently. It may be a sign of recovery from the grief of perinatal loss, in the same way as remarriage may be a sign of adjustment to being widowed (Littlewood, 1992). It may be suggested that the wish for another pregnancy may be a growth-promoting affirmation of life. There is, however, a dearth of research evidence to support this positive interpretation.

Urgency and grieving

The more usual view of the urgent desire for another pregnancy as a relatively early stage of grieving is demonstrated by research by Giles (1970) and by Wolff and colleagues (1970). Giles interviewed forty bereaved mothers in the early puerperium and shows their broad range of feelings about a future pregnancy. At one extreme, five mothers were doubtful of ever attempting another pregnancy, because their self-esteem was too low to allow them to contemplate success. At the opposite extreme was a similarly small group who were desperate to conceive again really quickly. This group of desperate women probably equate with a similar, but larger, group in Wolff's study. These researchers interviewed fifty bereaved mothers, also in the early postnatal period, but with a three-year follow-up, thus learning of their plans as well as their pregnancies. An immediate pregnancy was planned by 40 per cent of the mothers, but 50 per cent actually conceived within three years.

Wolff *et al.* (1970) regard these rapid pregnancies as examples of an immature response to the non-fulfilment of the women's fantasies of motherhood. Leon's psychotherapeutic approach (1990) interprets this reaction in terms of the mother's narcissism, self-esteem or self-love. Clearly the mother's self-image has been irrevocably damaged by her perception of her failure to give birth to a healthy baby. Leon argues that, for her, another, successful, pregnancy is the only route by which she is able to regain her equilibrium.

Deciding to begin another pregnancy

Making the decision about a future pregnancy may be influenced by a number of factors. Close family members as well as more casual acquaintances may urge the couple into parenthood. Or the woman's awareness of the ticking of her own biological clock may hurry her decision. On the other hand, fears of a similar outcome may deter the couple from another attempt.

The work of Wolff and colleagues shows us the large proportion, 50 per cent, of bereaved mothers who decide that the chance is not worth taking, and for half of these the decision was made irrevocable by sterilisation. Rowe *et al.* (1978) examined the association between having existing children and the decision to begin another pregnancy. This longitudinal study of twenty-six families grieving a perinatal death showed that those without living children were significantly more likely to embark on another pregnancy than those with children at home.

The timing of a future pregnancy is a source of concern; authors invariably consider the duration of the gap and often recommend a suitable time for the couple to plan a conception. The recommended time varies, but six months to one year is usual (Kargar, 1990; Kohner and Henley, 1992; Klaus and Kennell, 1982; Oglethorpe, 1989), but more recent literature is less prescriptive and may just suggest waiting for many months.

These prescriptions are reminiscent of the experience of Rose (1990), a psychotherapist who, on the death of her husband, listened to the advice and read the books and confidently expected her feelings to revert to normal one year after his death. She convinced herself of the truth of the twelve-month myth and that, on the magical date, her grief would disappear. She was shattered when she felt no better and eventually felt much worse on that date. Her experience warns us against being prescriptive about the duration of grief. The danger of such prescriptions is illustrated in the work of Rowe *et al.* (1978), who applied the label 'morbid grief' to parents who were still grieving twelve to twenty months after perinatal bereavement. The need to avoid fixed time periods is endorsed by Lewis and Bourne (1989) who refute the implication that longer grief is automatically abnormal grief, suggesting that we should look at the person rather than the calendar before labelling grief 'abnormal'.

The reasons for waiting are discussed by Kowalski (1987) and Oakley *et al.* (1984), who distinguish the physiological and the psychological factors. They conclude that the mother's body is likely to be ready within three to six months, but her emotional state may need at least twelve months to recover. Without recommending a time, Lewis and Page (1978) demonstrate the dangers of the mother becoming pregnant quickly after losing a baby and, hence, the reason for the importance which is attached to both the advice and the gap. In a case-study, a mother's inability to care for or relate to her healthy newborn daughter threatened the baby's survival. These psychotherapists attributed the mother's difficulty to her failure to mourn her stillborn first baby, who was born twelve months before his sister. By confronting the mother with her recollections of the first birth, the therapists forced her to begin the grieving which she had avoided, as evidenced by her second pregnancy. These authors regard a speedy pregnancy as evading the painfully difficult mourning of a perinatal death. Hence, the advice to wait.

The effect of pregnancy on grieving is said to derive from the incompatibility of these two processes in one person. Pregnancy eradicates grief, but the effect is not permanent, leaving the possibility that grief may reappear after the pregnancy ends (Lewis and Bourne, 1989).

One of the reasons for the incompatibility of grief and pregnancy relates to the need, in both, for the mother to adopt a particular mental stance to complete her emotional task, as both involve sorting out inevitable ambivalent feelings (Lewis, 1979b). When grieving, she focuses on her sorrow at ending her relationship with the dead person by recalling and working through her memories of that person. When pregnant she optimistically begins to establish her new relationship with her child, largely by fantasising about this new person and how she will relate to her or him. This is part of the process sometimes known as 'bonding'.

As well as the essentially diametrically opposed emotional approaches required, both processes are exclusive, in that they both prevent other emotional work being effectively completed simultaneously. Lewis and Bourne (1989) draw a picture of the mother's 'inner world' to explain this exclusivity; were it possible, this world would be inhabited by the dead baby she is grieving and the new baby she is starting to love. The internalisation of the images of the two babies simultaneously is prevented by the mother's fear that the new baby will be harmed by such close proximity to the dead baby. She, thus, blocks or unconsciously calls a halt to her grieving, which may be resumed either when her anxieties about her unseen new baby are dealt with or possibly at some other unpredictable future time. Lewis (1979b) alerts us to the risk that this incomplete mourning may reappear in a pathological form, activated by unforeseen events.

It is apparent that a new pregnancy will deprive the mother of both time and space for grieving her lost baby (Bourne and Lewis, 1984). The long-term implications are difficult to foresee, but we may be certain that a mother who hurries, or is hurried, into another pregnancy may find her experience unpleasant or even traumatic.

This decidedly pessimistic psychoanalytical view of a hasty conception may be questioned. A midwife with experience of being in this position argues the inaccuracy of this interpretation. Bower (1995) suggests, on the basis of her experience, that: 'a subsequent pregnancy is an integral and important part of the grieving process. The emotions which must be confronted during another childbearing experience are unique and will be felt whether they occur three months or three years after the original loss' (1995: 119–20).

Conceiving and being pregnant

When the bereaved couple feel ready to embark on a pregnancy, their difficulties are far from over. In a retrospective epidemiological study, Vogel and Knox (1975) found that couples who had experienced perinatal or early infant death attempted to compensate for their loss by a rapid pregnancy. This resulted in a rise in the fertility rate of the sample in the year following bereavement. But this increase was not maintained, to the extent that over a five-year period there was a marked reduction in their fertility. Alongside this effective fall in fertility, their success in childbearing was further reduced by a tendency for deaths to recur.

This observation of impaired childbearing following loss has also been noted in the context of parents who have lost a child through Sudden Infant Death Syndrome (SIDS). The work of Mandell and Wolfe (1975) focused on subsequent pregnancies in forty-one couples bereaved by SIDS. Of the mothers, eight were keen to avoid pregnancy and used contraception. After one mother, who was pregnant when bereaved, gave birth prematurely, only thirteen mothers had no problems with conceiving and carrying the pregnancy. Ten mothers experienced their first ever miscarriage, two of whom were subsequently infertile. Among this previously fertile group, the next pregnancy took between fifteen months and seven years to conceive. These 'problem pregnancy' rates are clearly higher than the expected infertility and miscarriage rates.

On the basis of these data Mandell and Wolfe propose that grieving is a psychological state which lowers the couple's childbearing ability. This suggestion is endorsed by the work of Vogel and Knox, which indicates that grieving couples' attempts to enlarge their families are frustrated by lower long-term fertility and associated with poorer outcomes. The effect of psychological stress on fertility is well established (Bancroft, 1989). The effects of grief are less well known, though the pathologically oriented work of Fenster *et al.* (1997) indicates a seriously negative effect on male fertility. Thus, it seems that grief may have a similarly adverse effect on general fertility. Our care of grieving parents should include a warning that a, hopefully temporary, decline in their fertility may be expected.

In terms of actually being pregnant following perinatal loss, the work of Hense in Canada investigated the woman's entire childbearing experience (1994). Hense undertook a phenomenological study with a suitably small number of primary and a larger number of secondary informants. Hense's informants began by revisiting the guilt which they experienced after their baby was stillborn. This led to a fear that they would never be able to give birth to the child they hoped for. If another pregnancy happened speedily, the women soon became aware of the risk of giving birth to an 'anniversary baby' (see page 90; Lewis and Page, 1978) and dreading birthdays.

The informants in Hense's sample assumed a paradoxical attitude towards 'replacing' the baby who was lost (see 'The replacement child syndrome', page 204). Both Hense and the women themselves explicitly discussed 'replacement' (1994: 171), but they were resentful when another person suggested this motivation for a speedy conception: 'I remember one of the nurses . . . Her advice was "Try to have another child as soon as possible to fill that void" ' (Lucy, 1994: 171). When the pregnancy was achieved and confirmed, the concept of replacement continued, but became more complex. The women found difficulty distinguishing between the two pregnancies and, hence, the two babies: 'Even waiting the length of time I did [four months] sometimes . . . it feels like I have been pregnant all along now. Just continuing on' (Sarah, 1994: 172). In order to assist the distinction between the babies, the women hoped that the baby they were carrying would be a different gender: 'I wanted him to be a girl so badly because I didn't want to be reminded of our first child' (Marie, 1994: 173). One mother, however, was so happy with this lack of distinction that she used the same name for her second child (see 'The name of the dead child', page 205): 'And there is another Samuel Brian really but it is two babies' (Carla, 1994: 173). The fear that the stillbirth might recur continued to haunt the woman throughout her pregnancy, as has been found also by Côté-Arsenault and Morrison-Beedy (2001). This fear resulted in the woman being unprepared to commit herself emotionally by becoming attached to her second unborn baby. This refusal to 'bond' was assisted by the woman concealing her pregnancy from people who might try to become, and to make her become, more involved. The fear of recurrence further led the woman to seek to protect her unborn child from any perceived danger: 'My main project every day was to keep watching my diet and nutrition and blood sugar' (Helen, 1994: 181). The women did recognise, though, that such extreme care of their health may have been counterproductive, in that it exposed the baby to an unhealthy level of stress, which was in itself regarded as harmful. The women sought reassurance of the baby's well-being from the full battery of prenatal tests, but sensibly drew the line at repeating tests unnecessarily.

After the baby was born alive and well, many of the woman's anxieties were not resolved, but continued in a slightly modified form. These included the problem of accepting the child as a separate individual and deciding what emotional commitment and tangible investment should be made for this new baby.

Thus, Hense's research shows clearly that the birth of a stillborn baby has serious consequences in any future pregnancy. These findings are endorsed by quantitative studies which have shown that depression levels are higher in women who have previously given birth to a stillborn baby (Armstrong, 2002) and particularly if they conceive within one year of the birth (Hughes *et al.*, 1999).

Care in a subsequent pregnancy

In a future pregnancy it will be necessary to regard the mother as high-risk. This applies especially if the reasons for the death have not been identified, but the increased likelihood of a poor outcome puts this mother in need of particularly vigilant care.

The demands on the woman who becomes pregnant after a perinatal loss are hugely increased. Superimposed on all the physical and psychological tasks which pregnancy requires, she has not only the demands of the additional investigations, but she also has the illness tasks involved in adapting to the patient role.

To avoid memories of sadness and loss, Kargar (1990) suggests that the mother's antenatal care should be provided 'well away from the hospital'. Whether such out-of-hospital care is consistent with the vigilant care which is required for this mother is questionable, but her intensive support would be more easily offered in an out-of-hospital setting.

The value of concentrated support, without high-tech interventions, during pregnancy has been shown to increase the rate of successful pregnancies in couples with a poor childbearing history (Stray-Pedersen and Stray-Pedersen, 1984). Similarly, the qualitative study by Côté-Arsenault and Freije (2004) in the USA indicates that 'Pregnancy After Loss' support groups were very acceptable to couples attending them.

The value of more intensive antenatal care is endorsed by the recommendation that time should be made available for this mother to talk and ask questions about the current pregnancy as well as the previous unsuccessful one (Lewis and Bourne, 1989; Sherr, 1989). Contemplating support during pregnancy leads to the question of whether more intensive care in the form of counselling or psychotherapy has any advantages over the support already described. Oglethorpe (1989) states that analytical psychotherapy may be technically difficult at this time, has particular hazards and carries no marked benefits (Apprey, 1987).

After the birth

The arrival of the new baby may resurrect in the mother many of the feelings associated with the loss of her previous baby:

JOSIE: In the case of the bereaved mother the baby is dead and it is all over, that is until she has a future pregnancy and all the memories will come flooding back.

If the mother's grieving is incomplete, she may suppress her strong feelings of loss which may continue to blank out her emotions (Lewis, 1979b). The difficulty for the mother in establishing a relationship with a new baby while still grieving the loss of a previous one has been mentioned already. This carries the risk that her feelings of affection for her new baby will be diminished and her relationship with her impaired.

As discussed already, delayed grieving is a response which may happen if a pregnancy quickly follows perinatal death (Sherr, 1989). The problems of an over-hasty conception are detailed in a case-study (Lewis and Page, 1978) in which the second child was born twelve months after her stillborn brother, making her an 'anniversary baby'. For anyone who has been bereaved, anniversaries are difficult, but the conflict between celebrating a birth at the same time as recalling the 'death-day' engenders bewilderment in the parents. Avoidance of an anniversary birth constitutes a further reason for delaying the next conception. It is necessary to be vigilant for these coincidences, either prospectively or retrospectively, in order to help the parents to open up and share any underlying feelings.

The replacement child syndrome

The reality of this syndrome has been advanced by psychologists and psychoanalysts, but has been questioned by more recent work. I address the evidence in favour of the existence of replacement child syndrome first. Oglethorpe (1989) defines a replacement child as either one who is specifically conceived to replace one who has died or a child forced by its family into this role. The term, however, tends to be used rather loosely to describe any child who is born soon after a loss or disappointment.

In their groundbreaking paper on this topic, Cain and Cain (1964) drew on their experience of six families who had suddenly lost a mature child through illness or accident. The severe psychiatric morbidity in, usually, the bereaved mother signified unresolved grief, which resulted in the, albeit hesitant, decision to replace the lost child.

Cain and Cain describe the birth of a child into an environment totally bound up with the memory of the dead child. The parents were more mature, possibly in their 40s, and their expectation was hardly for an infant, as they were seeking a replacement for an older child. The identification of the new child with its dead sibling was overpowering and constant comparisons were made. Unfortunately for the replacement child, the dead sibling was 'hyperidealised' quite unrealistically.

In my research on relinquishment, Ursula, contemplating a 'replacement child', recognised the risk of 'idealising' the one who was relinquished, with the potential for trauma:

URSULA: Another problem is that he is the perfect child. He has no bad points and will always be quite unique to me. Because when I first saw him he was perfect at his birth and every time I saw him after that he was being good. I s'pose that it's like meeting anybody for the first time. You don't get to know any of their bad points until you've met them a few times.

Cain and Cain focus on the prevalent psychiatric disturbances found among the replacement children, whose difficulties do not diminish as they grow older. These researchers consider the family pathology engendered by well-meaning but ill-informed friends and professionals who had recommended 'having another'.

Whether this syndrome, derived from case-studies following the deaths of older children, is applicable to perinatal loss deserves consideration. Cain and Cain (1964) and Leon (1990) argue that the more limited investment in a fetus or neonate reduces the likelihood of such a severe reaction. But Bluglass (1980) has demonstrated, in the context of SIDS, that problems of a similar nature do occur after the deaths of relatively young babies. To apply this knowledge to practice, it is necessary to bear in mind that the risk of replacement child syndrome is thought to increase if the parents have no contact with or recollection of the dead baby (Leon, 1990).

These views of replacement child syndrome tend to regard childbearing in a reductionist way, as a reactive process. The opposite point of view is advanced by Grout and Romanoff (2000) whose qualitative research demonstrates that family-building occurs in a more proactive way. The main activity of grieving, these authors maintain, comprises the reconstruction of meanings. In this way family relationships and family members' roles change and are changed to accommodate the new reality. Thus, parents' expectations, though decided at an early stage, are adjusted if a child is lost and her memory is integrated into the family, rather than being obliterated as the psychologists and psychoanalysts (above) envisage. The other family members are likely to continue to recognise the brief existence of the child who died and to acknowledge its effect on the dynamics of the family. Thus, rather than replacement, as the name of this syndrome suggests, the family processes continue to feature adaptation and reconstruction.

The name of the dead child

The name of the dead child has only recently attracted concern, because it acknowledges the reality and the individuality of the child. In thinking about any subsequent pregnancy the name assumes even greater significance; this is because the re-use of the same or a similar first name for a later child is considered indicative of pathological grief, that is, replacement child syndrome, and may forewarn of attendant risks. In their paper on this syndrome, Cain and Cain (1964) recount the confusion which the bereaved parents in their sample showed, by mistakenly addressing the replacement child by the name of the dead sibling. They suggest that this situation is aggravated by using a similar-sounding name, perhaps gender-adjusted, for the replacement child. The underlying problem is spelt out by Bourne and Lewis (1984):

> We believe it something of a disaster for the next baby to be saddled with the name formerly intended for the one who died, adding to the

danger that the new baby is only precariously differentiated from the dead one.

These authors go on to suggest that we, as health care providers, are ideally situated to prevent names being re-used in this way. These researchers are suitably wary of the damage experienced by a 'replacement child' and regard the name as an important indicator. Unfortunately, they regard the name as little more than a label, or perhaps a diagnostic tool. The true significance of the name is discussed by Raphael-Leff (1991) in terms of it being a 'live myth' which is bestowed upon the child. She regards the name as an attribution, rather than merely a label. It represents the parents' hopes and aspirations for their child. Although the name may appear to represent just a character in a soap opera or a pop singer, to the parents this may be the pinnacle of achievement and their ultimate hopes for their child. Raphael-Leff traces the use of different names according to the prevailing cultural and religious beliefs. The practice in the UK of using the same family name through the generations is becoming less common, although this certainly applied in my own family where my father and two brothers all chose to use the same name!

Thus, the name may be seen to represent desirable qualities with which the parents hope that the child will be blessed. This leads us to question whether it is really inappropriate to re-use a name simply because the person for whom it was intended has died. Connolly (1989) reports the practice in the west of Ireland of giving the same name to a sibling of a dead child. He maintains that this is acceptable because of what the name represents, regardless of whether it has been used previously. Similarly, one of Hense's informants re-used her dead baby's name (1994).

Summary

It is clear that embarking on another pregnancy after perinatal loss brings with it a range of hazards. For the mother, the pregnancy itself may be evidence of inadequate grieving, with the likelihood of that grieving being resurrected at some unpredictable future time. For the child the chances of, first, being conceived and, second, surviving the perinatal period are reduced. In the event of replacement child syndrome, the risk of psychological trauma to the child/person is infinite.

The original reason for the conception of the child who was lost is not affected by the loss of that child. The need for a child, for whatever reason, still pertains within the family; so the next child, if there is one, should not necessarily be regarded as a replacement, but as a wanted, child.

Research evidence suggests that, if necessary, appropriate interventions are available to help the mother to achieve success in both childbearing and psychological terms. Thus, our concerns for the welfare of the family and a subsequent child may not always be justified. In the event of inappropriate grief responses our interventions to help the family are able to prevent morbidity.

Conclusion

Benefits and meanings

Tread softly because you tread on my dreams.
(W. B. Yeats, 1899)

To conclude, I draw out two interrelated themes which have emerged repeatedly throughout this book. Although we tend to think automatically of the tragic nature of perinatal loss, there may be another side to this tragedy, perhaps even positive aspects. An example is the loving relationship which is the precursor to grief, on which I focused in the early chapters; included with this should be the personal growth and development which follows grief.

Findings of personal growth through increased self-knowledge emerged from a study of mothers' experience of miscarriage (Bansen and Stevens, 1992), together with heightened perceptions of both the joys and trauma of life, which was associated with an increased sense of responsibility. This manifested itself in the mother assuming a greater degree of control over her life and health.

These positive aspects are similar to those which may be found in the strengthening of parental relationships after the death of a child. An increased awareness of each other's priorities and recognition of their own strength may be associated with a new sensitivity to both the feelings and the pain of others. Researchers have identified benefits in terms of improved communication between bereaved parents (Helmrath and Steinitz, 1978). Those who were able to share their feelings increased their mutual trust and felt that this was essential to the resolution of their grief. The couples also thought that the quality of their relationship had improved and perceived the loss of their baby as an opportunity for personal growth.

The experience of loss may, in more general terms, provide a stimulus for major creative efforts. This may happen through the bereaved person being forced to reappraise their situation or simply through the space left by the absence of the loved one. In the same way, the experience of perinatal loss has served to stimulate creativity in women such as Mary Shelley, Anais Nin and Harriet Beecher Stowe. In Chapter 9, I showed how childhood grief later found artistic expression in the work of Edvard Munch.

The extent to which these positive aspects affect the feelings of loss depends on the unique meaning which is attributed to the loss. The attribution of meaning is closely linked with the cultural context, for example the concept of the 'good death' mentioned in Chapter 1. In the Western hemisphere, grieving a death is increasingly being regarded as a psychological condition rather than having physical connotations. In spite of this, in many cultures the dead body is still of major significance. So too, though, are the bodies of those who remain, as they may represent aspects of the loss. Examples may be found in analogies of grief as a limb or other body part being missing, or even the familiar broken heart. Thus, the meaning of the loss may emerge in physical signs, symptoms and perceptions through the process of somatisation.

The meaning which the mother attaches to her experience, though, may be less easy to identify. It is inevitable that the meaning which the pregnancy holds for her influences her grief. That meaning is highly individual and may include elements ranging from narcissistic self-absorption to a search for recognition of her adulthood. We must be wary of regarding perinatal loss as the loss of a baby and nothing more. In the event of such a loss we must take account of a wide range of personal and relational implications and accept that, additionally, there will be some which are not known to anyone but the grieving parents and, perhaps, not even to them. The poem by Yeats, the final line of which heads this chapter, was written in a very different context. It clearly shows, though, the fragility of meanings which, like dreams, may be unknown to the person herself.

An absence of meaning for the loss and, possibly, for life itself features in the later stages of acute grief (Parkes, 1976). The interpretation of her loss determines the extent to which the mother feels able to control her situation, which has implications for our care. As carers we are able to help her find the meaning of her loss; an example is how we provide opportunities and allow her space to fathom the unique meaning of her loss. The family has been shown to be similarly better able to cope if it is able to find meaning (Cook and Oltjenbruns, 1989).

As is so often the case, we are able to learn from the example of children, in whom the dynamic process by which the meaning of loss develops as the child sibling matures is clearly apparent. This is partly due to the child openly and uninhibitedly searching for meaning, whereas in adults that search is more secretive. In the same way as the meaning of her pregnancy determines her grief if the pregnancy is lost, so too the meaning the mother attributes to her child influences her response if her child has a disability.

While her reaction to her loss is influenced by a wide range of unknown factors, including the meaning of her loss, so too is her behaviour. The mother's response is affected by personal and cultural experiences which we may not share and which, to us, make her behaviour meaningless. But to her these behaviours and rituals are imbued with a profound significance, deserving our respect.

We are warned to avoid assumptions, especially of the meaning of the pregnancy and its loss (Worden, 2003). While we may be safer assuming that her loss constitutes an incapacitating tragedy, we should be prepared for and accepting of other reactions. The assumptions of some, such as the gurus who trivialise miscarriage with accusations of it being 'magnified into a catastrophe' (Bourne and Lewis, 1991), serve only to reinforce Worden's warning.

As I have suggested already, the benefits of loss and grief are not immediately obvious. The ideas of Marris (1986) provide a helpful framework which illuminate the enduring benefits of the pain which we all know. Marris believes that we create 'structures of meaning', which comprise an organised set of perceptions and beliefs which help us to make sense of our experiences in relation to the context in which they happen. Our structures of meaning preserve an element of continuity, by providing a system through which we are able to integrate new experiences into an existing mental framework. This is clearly essential when continuity is as fundamentally threatened as it is during perinatal bereavement. Marris's hypothesis suggests that grief constitutes a reaction to the disintegration of the structure of meaning associated with the lost relationship. Thus, grief comprises efforts to transform the meaning of the relationship to allow continuity to be restored. For these reasons, some degree of discomfort or distress is an inevitable consequence of loss. It needs to be perceived as a constructive, rather than just an inevitable, experience which helps us to adapt to maintain the continuity of life (Craig, 1977).

In this book I began by looking at the meanings of the words commonly used when talking about loss. To close, I have drawn together the recurring themes of the meaning of the loss itself and the long-term and intrinsic benefits of grief.

Appendix 1

Mysterious discovery: children's cemetery has been found in Astypalaia

Was it a maternity clinic or a sanctuary in which people offered up their dead babies in Astypalaia in ancient times? Was it a place where the gods were worshipped or just a cemetery, this place discovered on an island in the Aegean? Archaeological research is trying to answer these questions after this unique discovery.

The research started 5 years ago after a request by some local people to build houses in that area. Subsequently, the 22nd Ephorate of Prehistoric and Classical Antiquities discovered 150 vessels during a first excavation. Up to now, 1800 burials in large pottery vessels (amphorae) have been discovered. More burials are expected to be revealed as the excavation proceeds. It is obvious that the place was a cemetery. However, the necropolis of the ancient town of the island was detected on a hill named Katsalos, opposite the Venetian castle. Katsalos was used from the Late Geometric period to Roman times. After the initial excavation the 22nd Ephorate collaborated with the anthropology department of University College London, with Dr Hillson in charge.

Most of the 500 child skeletons found belong to newborn babies, with the exception of two cases of twins, three cases of children at the age of three and two of children at the age of five. Archaeologists wonder why so many babies were buried at that place. An epigraph at the museum of Astypalaia may provide us with an answer. It refers to the Goddess of Diana. Diana was worshipped as the goddess of labour, among other things. According to mythology, she was the first to be delivered by Leto and she was the midwife of her brother Apollo. Archaeologists suspect that there was a sanctuary of Diana in Astypalaia and that people from neighbouring islands offered her their dead babies. According to another theory, a maternity clinic may have existed there with a doctor or midwives helping women in labour; the great number of baby burials could be explained by the high mortality of those years.

(Anagnostou, 2004)

Appendix 2
My youngest brother

It's hard to remember the precise details of what happened when. I was ten, almost fifty years ago. I had been around when Mummy had my younger brother, so I knew all about it. I was able to help her get things ready during the winter. We got the cot out. She knitted vests. We cleaned her bedroom so that it would be OK for the midwife, Nurse Pearce, when she came for the birth. Everybody said how good I was – a proper little midwife!

Funny that.

Nothing happened.

I knew that when someone was going to have a baby, they have a baby. But Mummy didn't.

I remember Mummy having to stay in bed. I still don't know why.

Then things disappeared. The cot was put away. The knitting stopped.

Everybody was very nice to me. But nobody told me anything. It was obvious I wasn't supposed to ask. So I didn't. They probably thought I'd forgotten about the baby.

When pancake day came round we were sent to the doctor's house and his wife cooked our dinner. It was meant to be a treat. Then I was sent to stay with my Aunt in Wales for Easter.

One day, some time later, Daddy came to school. This was quite unheard of. I went outside to see him. It wasn't winter any more. He sat on the steps. He'd brought me a new windcheater. I didn't know why, but it was nice.

At the end of school my elder sister collected me to go shopping. She was a nurse and knew a lot about things.

When we went into Mrs Martin's shop, she asked how Mummy was. My sister said she'd had a baby boy, but he was born dead. Because I knew by then I wasn't supposed to talk about it, I didn't say anything.

Nobody said anything to me. I suppose I was too young to understand. I decided that his name was Michael.

Years later, a short while before Daddy died, he told me how sorry he was that the baby had died. He'd have liked another boy.

What was Michael like? Was he formed properly? Is he buried somewhere? I wish I knew.

Although I've never been told anything about him, I learned a lot from Michael.

I learned that there are some things that you just do not talk about.

Is it because it doesn't matter when someone dies? It seemed like that. Nobody bothered. Nobody cried.

Or is it because dying is too awful to speak about? It takes a long time to learn that some things are better talked about.

Or is it that babies don't matter? We were a big family. What does one child matter?

Or perhaps I was told about it – well half-told when Mrs Martin was told. But I was also being protected by not being told.

I'm sure they all thought it was for the best.

(A bereaved sibling)

References

Adams, M. and Prince, J. (1990) Care of the grieving parent with special reference to stillbirth, in Alexander, J., Levy, V. and Roch, S. (eds), *Post Natal Care: A Research-based Approach*, Ch. 7, pp. 108–24. London: Macmillan.

Adams, R. (1990) *Self-help, Social Work and Empowerment*. Basingstoke/London: Macmillan Education.

Adams, R. (1996) *Social Work and Empowerment*, 2nd edn. Basingstoke: Macmillan.

Adamsen, L. Rasmussen, J.M. (2001) Sociological perspectives on self-help groups: reflections on conceptualization and social processes, *Journal of Advanced Nursing*, 35:6, pp. 909–17.

Adshead, G. and Dickenson, D. (1993) Why do doctors and nurses disagree?, in Dickenson, D. and Johnson, M. *Death, Dying and Bereavement*. London: OU/Sage.

Allingham, M. (1952) *Tiger in the Smoke*. London: Chatto & Windus.

Anagnostou, D. (2004) Mysterious discovery: children's cemetery has been found in Astypalaia, *Eleutherotypia*, 12 July 2004.

Anderson, G.C., Moore, E., Hepworth, J. and Bergman, N. (2004) Early skin-to-skin contact for mothers and their healthy newborn infants (Cochrane Review), in *The Cochrane Library*, Issue 3. Chichester, UK: John Wiley.

Ankum, W.M., Wieringa-de Waard, M. and Bindels, P.J.E. (2001) Management of spontaneous miscarriage in the first trimester: an example of putting informed shared decision-making into practice, *British Medical Journal*, 322:7298, pp. 1343–6.

Anon (1993) A cry for help, *Nursing Times*, 27 January, 89:4, pp. 29–30.

Apprey, M. (1987) Projective identification and maternal misconception in disturbed mothers, *British Journal of Psychotherapy*, 4, pp. 5–22.

Armstrong, D.S. (2002) Emotional distress and prenatal attachment in pregnancy after perinatal loss, *Journal of Nursing Scholarship*, 34:4, pp. 339–45.

Ashmore, R. and Banks, D. (2001) Patterns of self-disclosure among mental health nursing students, *Nurse Education Today*, 21:1, pp. 48–57.

Awoonor-Renner, S. (2000) I desperately needed to see my son, Ch. 54, p. 347 in Dickenson, D., Johnson, M. and Katz, J.S. (eds), *Death, Dying and Bereavement*, 2nd edn. London: Open University Press/Sage.

Ayers, S. Pickering, A.D. (2001) Do women get posttraumatic stress disorder as a result of childbirth? A prospective study of incidence, *Birth*, 28:2, pp. 111–18.

Baggaley, S. (1993) Personal communication.

Bailey, R. and Clarke, M. (1991) *Stress and Coping in Nursing*. London: Chapman & Hall.

Bancroft, J.H.J. (1989) *Human Sexuality and its Problems*. Edinburgh: Churchill Livingstone.

Bansen, S.S. and Stevens, H.A. (1992) Women's experience of miscarriage in early pregnancy, *Journal of Nurse Midwifery*, March–April, 37:2, pp. 84–90.

Barker, J. (1983) Volunteer bereavement counselling schemes, Age Concern Research Unit.

Barth, A., Egger, A. Hladschik-Hermer, B. and Kropiunigg, U. (2004) Tränen im Krankenhaus – eine Bestandsaufnahme unter Arzten, Pflegepersonal und Medizinstudenten [Shedding tears in hospitals – a survey of medical staff and students], *Psychotherapie, Psychosomatik, Medizinische Psychologie*, 54:5, pp. 194–7.

Becker, P.T., Grunwald, P.C., Moorman, J. and Stuhr, S. (1991) Outcomes of developmentally supportive Nursing care for VLBW infants, *Nursing Research*, 40:3, pp. 150–5.

Beech, B.L. (1998/9) Book review, *AIMS Journal*, 10:4, p. 21.

Begley, C. (2003) 'I cried . . . I had to . . .': student midwives' experiences of stillbirth, miscarriage and neonatal death, *Evidence Based Midwifery*, 1:1, pp. 20–6.

Belcher, L. and St Lawrence, J. (2000) Women and HIV, Ch. 17, pp. 305–26 in Sherr, L. and St Lawrence, J.S. (eds) *Women, Health and the Mind*. Chichester: Wiley.

Bender, H. and Swan-Parente, A. (1983) Psychological and psychotherapeutic support of staff and parents in an intensive care baby unit, in Davis, J.A., Richards, M.P.M. and Roberton, N.R.C., *Parent–Baby Attachment in Premature Infants*. London: Croom Helm.

Benfield, D.G., Leib, S.A. and Reuter, J. (1976) Grief responses of parents after referral of the critically ill newborn to a regional center, *New England Journal of Medicine*, 294, pp. 975–8.

Benfield, D.G., Leib, S.A. and Vollman, J.H. (1978) Grief response of parents to neonatal death and parent participation in deciding care, *Pediatrics*, August, 62:2, pp. 171–6.

Bennett, C.C., Lal, M.K., Field, D.J. and Wilkinson, A.R. (2002) Maternal morbidity and pregnancy outcome in a cohort of mothers transferred out of perinatal centres during a national census, *British Journal of Obstetrics and Gynaecology*, 109:6, pp. 663–6.

Beutel, M., Willner, H., Deckardt, R., von Rad, M. and Weiner, H. (1996) Similarities and differences in couples' grief reactions following a miscarriage: results from a longitudinal study, *Journal of Psychosomatic Research*, 4:3, pp. 245–523.

Bewley, C. (1993) The midwife's role in pregnancy termination, *Nursing Standard*, 8:12, pp. 25–8.

Bluglass, K. (1980) Psychiatric morbidity after cot death, *Practitioner*, 224, pp. 533–9.

Bolton, S.C. (2000) Who cares? Offering emotion work as a 'gift' in the nursing labour process, *Journal of Advanced Nursing*, 32:3, pp. 580–6.

Bond, M. (1986) *Stress and Self-Awareness: A Guide for Nurses*. London: Heinemann.

Boris, N.W., Aoki, Y. and Zeanah, C.H. (1999) The development of infant–parent attachment: considerations for assessment, *Infants and Young Children*, 11:4, pp. 1–10.

Bott, J. (2000) Clinical. HIV and women: health and childbearing issues, *British Journal of Midwifery*, 8:1, pp. 15–9.

Bouchier, P., Lambert, L. and Triseliotis, J. (1991) *Parting with a Child for Adoption: The Mother's Perspective*, Discussion Series, 14. London: British Agencies for Adoption and Fostering.

Bourne, S. (1968) The psychological effects of stillbirth on women and their doctors, *Journal of Royal College of General Practitioners*, 16, pp. 103–12.

Bourne, S. (1979) Coping with perinatal death, *Midwife, Health Visitor and Community Nurse*, February, pp. 59, 62.

Bourne, S. and Lewis, E. (1984) Pregnancy after stillbirth or neonatal death, *Lancet*, July, 7:2, pp. 31–3.

Bourne, S. and Lewis, E. (1991) Perinatal bereavement: a milestone and some new dangers, *British Medical Journal*, 302, pp. 1167–8.

Bower, H. (1995) Loss and bereavement in childbearing, *MIDIRS*, 5:1, pp. 119–20.

Bowlby, J. (1958) The nature of the child's tie to his mother, *International Journal of Psychoanalysis*, 30, p. 350.

Bowlby, J. (1961) Processes of mourning, *International Journal of Psychoanalysis*, 44, p. 317.

Bowlby, J. (1977) The making and breaking of affectional bonds I and II, *British Journal of Psychiatry*, 130, pp. 201–10, 421–31.

Bowlby, J. (1984) The making and breaking of affectional bonds, in BAAF (ed.), *Working with Children*. London: BAAF.

Bowlby, J. (1990) *The Making and Breaking of Affectional Bonds*. London: Routledge.

Boyle, F.M. (1997) *Mothers Bereaved by Stillbirth, Neonatal Death or Sudden Infant Death Syndrome*. Aldershot: Ashgate.

Bradshaw, Z. and Slade, P. (2003) The effects of induced abortion on emotional experiences and relationships: a critical review of the literature, *Clinical Psychology Review*, 23:7, pp. 929–58.

Brazelton, T.B. (1973) *Neonatal Behavioral Assessment Scale*. London: SIMP.

Brocklehurst, P. (2004) Interventions for reducing the risk of mother-to-child transmission of HIV infection (Cochrane Review), in *The Cochrane Library*, Issue 2. Chichester, UK: John Wiley.

Brocklehurst, P. and French, R. (1998) The association between maternal HIV infection and perinatal outcome: a systematic review of the literature and meta-analysis, *British Journal of Obstetrics and Gynaecology*, 105:8, pp. 836–48.

Brubaker, T.H. (1987) *Aging, Health and Family: Long-term Care*. Newbury Park, Calif.: London: Sage.

Bryan, E. (1992) *Twins and Higher Multiple Births: A Guide to their Nature and Nurture*. London: Edward Arnold.

Bryan, E.M. (1999) Twins, Ch. 25, pp. 409–16 in Rennie, J.M. and Roberton, N.R.C. (2002) *A Manual of Neonatal Intensive Care*, 4th edn. London: Arnold.

Buckman, R. (2000) Communication in palliative care: a practical guide, Ch. 26, pp. 146–73, in Dickenson, D., Johnson, M. and Katz, J.S. (eds), *Death, Dying and Bereavement*. London: Sage.

Burnard, P. and Morrison, P. (1991) Client-centred counselling: a study of nurses' attitudes, *Nurse Education Today*, April, 11:2, pp. 104–9.

Burns, D. and Taylor, M. (1998) *Mutual Aid and Self-help: Coping Strategies for Excluded Communities*. Bristol: Policy Press.

Cahill, J. (1998) Patients' perceptions of bedside handovers, *Journal of Clinical Nursing*, 7:4, pp. 351–9.

Cain, A.C. and Cain, B.S. (1964) On replacing a child, *Journal of the American Academy of Child Psychiatry*, 3, pp. 433–56.

Callan, V.J. and Hennessy, J.F. (1989) Psychological adjustment to infertility: a unique comparison of two groups of infertile women, mothers and women childless by choice, *Journal of Reproductive and Infant Psychology*, 7:2, pp. 105–12.

Cameron, J. and Parkes, C.M. (1983) Terminal care: evaluation of effects on surviving family of care before and after bereavement, *Postgraduate Medical Journal*, 59, pp. 73–8.

Campbell, A.V. (1979) The meaning of death and ministry to the dying, in Doyle, D. (ed.), *Terminal Care*. Edinburgh: Churchill Livingstone.

Campbell, J. (1733) Campbell of Barcaldine Papers. National Archives of Scotland GD170/793.

Campbell, T. and Bernhardt, S. (2003) Factors that contribute to women declining antenatal HIV testing, *Health Care for Women International*, 24:6, pp. 544–51.

Caplan, G. (1961) *An approach to community mental health*. London: Tavistock.

Carlisle, C., Baker, G.A., Riley, M. and Dewey, M. (1994) Stress in midwifery: a comparison of midwives and nurses using the Work Environment Scale, *International Journal of Nursing Studies*, 31:1, pp. 13–22.

Carter, D. (1991) Quantitative research, in Cormack, D., *The Research Process in Nursing*, 2nd edn. London: Blackwell Scientific.

Carter, J.P. (2003) Pre-personality pregnancy losses: miscarriages, stillbirths and abortions, in Bryant, C.D. (ed.), *Handbook of Death and Dying*, p. 264. Thousand Oaks, Calif.: Sage.

Cecil, R. (1996) Introduction: an insignificant event?, in Cecil, R. (ed.), *The Anthropology of Pregnancy Loss*. Oxford: Berg.

Chalmers, I. (1993) Effective care in midwifery: research, the professions and the public, *Midwives Chronicle*, January, 106:1260, pp. 3–13.

Chambers, H.M. and Chan, F.Y. (2004) Support for women/families after perinatal death (Cochrane Review), in *The Cochrane Library*, Issue 3, Chichester, UK: John Wiley.

Chapman, R.R. (2003) Endangering safe motherhood in Mozambique: prenatal care as pregnancy risk, *Social Science and Medicine*, 57:2, pp. 355–74.

CHI (2004) *HIV Transmission through Breastfeeding: A Review of Available Evidence*, UNICEF, UNAIDS, WHO, UNFPA Center for HIV Information, http://www.unfpa.org/upload/lib_pub_file/276_filename_HIV_PREV_BF_GUIDE_ENG.pdf. Accessed July 2004.

Chiswick, M. (2001) Parents and end of life decisions in neonatal practice, *Archives of Disease in Childhood*, 85, F1–F3.

Chitty, L.S. Hunt, G.H., Moore, J. and Lobb, M.O. (1991) Effectiveness of routine ultrasonography in detecting fetal structural abnormalities in a low-risk population, *British Medical Journal*, 303:6811, pp. 1165–9.

Clark, G.T. (1991) To the edge of existence: living through grief, *Phenomenology and Pedagogy*, Fall Issue.

Cohan, D. (2003) *Perinatal HIV: Special Considerations*, International AIDS Society USA, Topics in HIV Medicine, http://www.iasusa.org/pub/topics/2003/issue6/nov_dec_2003.pdf. Accessed 14 July 2004.

Cole, A. (1993) Vital support, *Nursing Times*, 31 March, 89:13, pp. 16–17.

Conde-Agudelo, A., Diaz-Rossello, J.L. and Belizan, J.M. (2004) Kangaroo mother care to reduce morbidity and mortality in low birthweight infants (Cochrane Review), in *The Cochrane Library*, Issue 3. Chichester, UK: John Wiley.

Conduit, E. (1995) *The Body under Stress*. Hove: Lawrence Erlbaum Associates.

Connolly, K.D. (1989) Factors affecting grief following pregnancy loss. 9th

International Congress of Psychosomatic Obstetrics and Gynaecology, Amsterdam.

Cook, A.S. and Oltjenbruns, K.A. (1989) *Dying and Grieving: Life-span and Family Perspectives*. New York: Holt, Rinehart and Winston.

Cook, A.S and Dworkin, D.S. (1992) *Helping the Bereaved: Therapeutic Interventions for Children, Adolescents and Adults*. New York: Basic Books.

Cooke, P. (1990) Sudden maternal death and its effects on the family. London Thames Valley University, Unpublished course paper.

Cooper, J.D (1980) Parental reactions to stillbirth, *British Journal of Social Work*, 10:1, pp. 55–69.

Costello, J. (2001) Nursing older dying patients: findings from an ethnographic study of death and dying in elderly care wards, *Journal of Advanced Nursing*, 35:1, pp. 59–68.

Côté-Arsenault, D. and Dombeck, M.B. (2001) Maternal assignment of fetal person-hood to a previous pregnancy loss: relationship to anxiety in the current pregnancy, *Health Care for Women International*, 22:7, pp. 649–65.

Côté-Arsenault, D. and Morrison-Beedy, D. (2001) Women's voices reflecting changed expectations for pregnancy after perinatal loss, *Journal of Nursing Scholarship*, Third Quarter, 33:3, pp. 239–44.

Côté-Arsenault, D. and Freije, M.M. (2004) Support groups helping women through pregnancies after loss, *Western Journal of Nursing Research*, 26:6, pp. 650–70.

Coutsoudis, A., Pillay, K., Kuhn, L., Spooner E., Tsai, W.Y. and Coovadia, H.M. (2001) Method of feeding and transmission of HIV-1 from mothers to children by 15 months of age: prospective cohort study from Durban, South Africa, *AIDS*, 15:3, pp. 379–87.

Cowles, K.V. (1996) Cultural perspectives of grief: an expanded concept analysis, *Journal of Advanced Nursing*, 23:2, pp. 287–94.

Craig, Y. (1977) The bereavement of parents and their search for meaning, *British Journal of Social Work*, 7:1, pp. 41–54.

Cudmore, J. (1996) Preventing PTSD in accident and emergency nursing: a review of the literature, *Nursing in Critical Care*, 1:3, pp. 120–6.

Cunningham, C.C, Morgan, P.A. and Mcgucken, R.B. (1984) Down's syndrome: is dissatisfaction with disclosure of diagnosis inevitable?, *Developmental Medicine and Child Neurology*, 26, pp. 33–9.

Cunningham-Burley, S. (1984) 'We don't talk about it': issues of gender and method in the portrayal of grandfatherhood, *Sociology*, 18:3, pp. 325–38.

Curtis, P. (2000) Midwives' attendances at stillbirths: an oral history account, *MIDIRS Midwifery Digest*, 10:4, pp. 526–30.

Danbury, H. (1996) *Bereavement Counselling Effectiveness: A Client-Opinion Study*, Aldershot: Avebury.

Darbyshire, P. (1992) Telling stories, telling moments, *Nursing Times*, 1 January, 88:1, pp. 22–4.

Davidson, G. (1977) Death of the wished-for child: a case-study, *Death Education*, 1, p. 265.

Davies, R. (2001) Emotion work in midwifery: a review of current knowledge, *Journal of Advanced Nursing*, 34:4, pp. 436–44.

Davis, D.L., Stewart, M. and Harmon, R.J. (1988) Perinatal loss: providing emotional support for bereaved parents, *Birth*, 15:4, pp. 242–6.

Davis, J.A. (1983) Ethical issues in neonatal intensive care, in Davis, J.A., Richards,

M.P.M. and Roberton, N.R.C., *Parent–Baby Attachment in Premature Infants*. London: Croom Helm.

Dean, R. (1997) Humor and laughter in palliative care, *Journal of Palliative Care*, 13:1, pp. 24–39.

del Valle, H. (2004) *Beyond the Burqa – Addressing the Causes of Maternal Mortality in Afghanistan*, http://www.fmreview.org/text/FMR/19/04.htm. Accessed 3 January 2005.

Denzin, N.K. and Lincoln, Y.S. (2000) *Handbook of Qualitative Research*, 2nd edn. London: Sage.

DeVries, R. (1996) The midwife's place: an international comparison of the status of midwives, Ch. 13, pp. 159–74 in Murray, S.F. (ed.), *Midwives and Safer Motherhood*. London: Mosby.

Diekelmann, N. (1992) Show some emotion, *Nursing Times*, 88:44, pp. 46–8.

DiMarco, M.A., Menke, E.M. and McNamara, T. (2001) Evaluating a support group for perinatal loss, *MCN: The American Journal of Maternal/Child Nursing*, 26:3, pp. 135–40.

DoH (2003) Families and post-mortems: a code of practice, forms and information leaflets, Department of Health, http://www.dh.gov.uk/PolicyAndGuidance/HealthAndSocialCareTopics/Tissue/TissueGeneralInformation/TissueGeneral Article/fs/en?CONTENT_ID=4002253&chk=pjRv4o. Accessed 20 July 2004.

Dor, J. (1977) An evaluation of the etiologic factors in therapy in 665 infertile couples, *Fertility and Sterility*, 28:7, pp. 718–22.

Dosanjh, S., Barnes, J. and Bhandari, M. (2001) Barriers to breaking bad news among medical and surgical residents, *Medical Education*, 35:3, pp. 197–205.

Douglas, J. (1992) Black women's health matters: putting black women on the research agenda, Ch. 2, p. 33, in Roberts, H. *Women's Health Matters*. London: Routledge.

Downs, J.C.U. (2003) The autopsy, in Bryant, C.D. (ed.), *Handbook of Death and Dying*, Part V, pp. 523–33. Thousand Oaks, Calif.: Sage.

Drever, J. (1964) *A Dictionary of Psychology*. London: Penguin.

Druery, K. (1992) Bereavement support in a maternity unit, *MIDIRS Midwifery Digest*, 2:2, pp. 223–5.

Dunlop, R.J. and Hockley, J.M. (1990) *Terminal Care Support Teams*. Oxford: Oxford University Press.

Dyer, M. (1992) Stillborn – still precious, *MIDIRS Midwifery Digest*, June, 2:2, pp. 341–4.

Dyregrov, A. (1988) The loss of a child: the sibling's perspective, in Kumar, R. and Brockington, N. (eds), *Motherhood and Mental Illness 2: Causes and Consequences*. London: Wright.

Dyregrov, A. (1991) *Grief in Children: A Handbook for Adults*. London: Kingsley.

Dyson, L. and While, A. (1998) The 'long shadow' of perinatal bereavement, *British Journal of Community Nursing*, 3:9, pp. 432–9.

Eley, S. (2003) Virtual methods. Exploring online storytelling and support groups, http://www.soc.surrey.ac.uk/virtualmethods/vmpapers/susan.htm. Accessed 3 September 2004.

Engel, G.C. (1961) Is grief a disease? A challenge for medical research, *Psychosomatic Medicine*, 23, pp. 18–22.

Evans, M.I., Hume, R.F., Yaron, Y., Kramer, R.L. and Johnson, M.P. (1998) Multifetal pregnancy reduction, Ch. 10 in Neilson, J.P. (ed.), *Bailliere's Clinical Obstetrics and Gynaecology*, 12:1, Multiple Pregnancy, pp. 147–60.

Everett, H. (1997) Aims in termination counselling, Paper presented at Pro-Choice Forum Conference 'Issues in pregnancy counselling: what do women need and want?', Oxford, May.

Ewigman, B., Green, J. and Lumley, J. (1993) Ultrasound during pregnancy: a discussion. Interview by Max Allen, *Birth*, 20:4, pp. 212–15.

Eysenbach, G. and Till, J.E. (2001) Information in practice. Ethical issues in qualitative research on Internet communities, *British Medical Journal*, 323:7321, pp. 1103–5.

Farrant, W. (1985) Who's for amniocentesis? The politics of prenatal screening, Ch. 7 in Homans, H. (ed.), *The Sexual Politics of Reproduction*. Aldershot: Gower.

Farrell, M., Ryan, S. and Langrick, B. (2001) 'Breaking bad news' within a paediatric setting: an evaluation report of a collaborative education workshop to support health professionals, *Journal of Advanced Nursing*, 36:6, pp. 765–75.

Fenster, L., Katz, D.F., Wyrobek, A.J., Pieper, C. Rempel, D.M., Oman, D. and Swan, S.H. (1997) Effects of psychological stress on human semen quality, *Journal of Andrology*, 18:2, pp. 194–202.

Ferri, E. (1975) Characteristics of motherless families, *British Journal of Social Work*, 3:1, pp. 91–100.

Fielding, N.G. and Lee, R.M. (1991) *Using Computers in Qualitative Research*. London: Sage.

Fisher, J. (2001) Harming and benefiting the dead, *Death Studies*, 25:7, pp. 557–68.

Forna, F. and Gülmezoglu, A.M. (2004) Surgical procedures to evacuate incomplete abortion (Cochrane Review), in *The Cochrane Library*, Issue 2, Chichester, UK: John Wiley.

Forrest, G. (1989) Care of the bereaved after perinatal death, in Chalmers, I., Enkin, M. and Keirse, M.J.N.C. (eds), *Effective Care in Pregnancy and Childbirth*, Vol 2. Oxford: Oxford University Press.

Forrest, G.C. (1983) Mourning perinatal death, in Davis, J.A., Richards, M.P.M. and Roberton, N.R.C. (eds), *Parent–Baby Attachment in Premature Infants*. London: Croom Helm.

Forrest, G.C. (1999) Handling perinatal death, Ch. 6, pp. 73–8, in Rennie, J.M. and Roberton, N.R.C. (eds), *Textbook of Neonatology*, 3rd edn. Edinburgh: Churchill Livingstone.

Forrest, G.C., Standish, E. and Baum, J.D. (1982) Support after perinatal death: a study of support and counselling after perinatal bereavement, *British Medical Journal*, 20 November, 285:6353, pp. 1475–9.

Foster, A. (1996) Perinatal bereavement: support for families and midwives, *Midwives*, 109:1303, pp. 218–19.

Frank, D.I. (1984) Counselling the infertile couple, *Journal of Psychosocial Nursing*, May, 22:5, pp. 17–23.

Fransen, L. (2003) The impact of inequality on the health of mothers, *Midwifery*, 19:2, pp. 79–81.

Freud, S. (1955) Case histories, in Strachey, J. (ed. and trans.), *The Standard Edition of the Complete Psychological Works of Sigmund Freud*, Vol. XIII, pp. 22–1810. London: Hogarth Press. Original publication 1893–95.

Freud, S. (1959) *Mourning and Melancholia Collected Papers*. New York: Basic Books. Original publication 1917.

Friedman, T. and Gath, D. (1989) The psychiatric consequences of spontaneous abortion, *British Journal of Psychiatry*, 155, pp. 810–13.

Garber, J. and Seligman, M.E.P. (1980) *Human Helplessness: Theory and Applications.* New York: Academic Press.

Gelles, R.J. (1995) *Contemporary Families: A Sociological View.* Thousand Oaks, Calif./London: Sage.

Giles, P.F.H. (1970) Reactions of women to perinatal death, *Australian and New Zealand Journal of Obstetrics and Gynaecology,* 10, pp. 207–10.

Glaser, B.G. and Strauss, A.L. (1965) *Awareness of Dying.* Chicago, Ill.: Aldine Publishing.

Gohlish, M.C. (1985) Stillbirth, *Midwife, Health Visitor and Community Nurse,* 21:1, p. 16.

Gorer, G. (1965) *Death, Grief and Mourning in Contemporary Britain.* London: Cresset Press.

Grace, J.T. (1989) Development of maternal–fetal attachment during pregnancy, *Nursing Research,* July/August, 38:4, pp. 228–32.

Gray, J.M. (ed. 1892) Memoirs of the life of Sir John Clerk of Penicuik, baronet, baron of the Exchequer, extracted by himself from his own journals, 1676–1755. Edinburgh: Printed at Edinburgh University Press by T. and A. Constable for the Scottish History Society.

Green, J.M. and Baston, H.A. (2003) Feeling in control during labor: concepts, correlates, and consequences, *Birth,* 30:4, pp. 235–47.

Green, J.M., Statham, H. and Snowdon, C. (1993) Women's knowledge of prenatal screening tests, *Journal of Reproductive and Infant Psychology,* 11:1, pp. 31–40.

Greig, C. (1998) A survey of information given during pregnancy by midwives to parents about neonatal unit care, whether or not the baby was likely to require such care, *Midwifery,* 14:1, pp. 54–60.

Greig, C. (2002) Prenatal preparation of parents for neonatal care: a comparative descriptive study. University of Edinburgh, Unpublished Ph.D. thesis.

Grout, L.A. and Romanoff, B.D. (2000) The myth of the replacement child: parents' stories and practices after perinatal death, *Death Studies,* 24:2, pp. 93–113.

Guillemin, J.H. and Holmstrom, L.L. (1986) *Mixed Blessings: Intensive Care for Newborns.* Oxford: Oxford University Press.

Harlow, H.F. and Harlow, M.K. (1966) Learning to love, *American Scientist,* 54, pp. 244–72.

Harmon, R.J., Glicken, A.D. and Siegel, R.E. (1984) Neonatal loss in the intensive care nursery: effects on maternal grieving and program for intervention, *Journal of the American Academy of Child Psychiatry,* 23, pp. 68–71.

Hayslip, B. and Hansson, R.O. (2003) Death awareness and adjustment across the life-span, in Bryant, C.D. (ed.), *Handbook of Death and Dying,* Vol. 1, Part IV, pp. 437–47. Thousand Oaks, Calif.: Sage.

Hearn, K. (2001) *The Saltonstall Family by David des Granges,* http://www.tate.org.uk/servlet/ViewWork?cgroupid=999999961&workid=3821&tabview=text&texttype=10. Accessed 31 December 2004.

Helmrath, T.A. and Steinitz, E.M. (1978) Death of an infant: parental grieving and the failure of social support, in Rando, T.A. (ed.), *Parental Loss of Child.* Champaign, Ill.: Research Press.

Hense, A.L. (1994) Livebirth following stillbirth, Ch. 5 in Field, P.A. and Marck, P.B. (eds), *Uncertain Motherhood: Negotiating the Risks of the Childbearing Years.* Thousand Oaks. Calif.: Sage.

Herbert, M. and Sluckin, A. (1985) A realistic look at mother–infant bonding, in

Chiswick, M.L. (ed.), *Recent Advances in Perinatal Medicine: 2*. Edinburgh: Churchill Livingstone.

Herkes, B. (2002) Professional issues. A bereavement counselling service for parents, part 2, *British Journal of Midwifery*, 10:3, pp. 135–9.

Hicks, C. (1992) Research in midwifery: are midwives their own worst enemies?, *Midwifery*, 8:1, pp. 12–18.

Hicks, C.M. (1996) *Undertaking Midwifery Research: A Basic Guide to Design and Analysis*. Edinburgh: Churchill Livingstone.

Hillhouse, J.J. and Adler, C.M. (1997) Investigating stress effect patterns in hospital staff nurses: results of a cluster analysis, *Social Science and Medicine*, 45:12, pp. 1781–8.

Hillson, S. (2002) Investigating ancient cemeteries on the island of Astypalaia, Greece, *Archaeology International*, 2001/2002, pp. 29–31.

Hingley, P. and Marks, R. (1991) A stressful occupation, *Nursing Times*, 87:25, pp. 63–6.

Hochschild, A.R. (1983) *The Managed Heart: Commercialization of Human Feeling*. Berkeley, Calif.: University of California Press.

Hockley, J. (1989) Caring for the dying in acute hospitals, *Nursing Times*, 27 September, 85:39, pp. 47–50.

Horsfall, A. (2001) Bereavement: tissues, tea and sympathy are not enough, *RCM Midwives Journal*, 4:2, pp. 54–7.

Houlbrooke, R.A. (1984) *The English Family 1450–1700*. London: Longman.

Houlbrooke, R.A. (1998) *Death, Religion, and the Family in England, 1480–1750*. Oxford: Clarendon Press.

House of Commons (1992) Health Committee Second Report, Maternity.

Howarth, G. and Leaman, O. (2001) *Encyclopedia of Death and Dying*. London: Routledge.

Hsu, M., Tseng, Y. and Kuo, L. (2002) Transforming loss: Taiwanese women's adaptation to stillbirth, *Journal of Advanced Nursing*, 40:4, pp. 387–95.

Hughes, P. (1986) Solitary or solitude: views on the management of bereaved mothers. University of Wales, Unpublished Dip.N. dissertation.

Hughes, P. (1987) The management of bereaved mothers: what is best?, *Midwives Chronicle*, August, 100:1195, pp. 226–9.

Hughes, P., Turton, P. and Evans, C.D. (1999) Stillbirth as risk factor for depression and anxiety in the subsequent pregnancy: cohort study, *British Medical Journal*, 318:7200, pp. 721–4.

Hughes, P., Turton, P., Hopper, E. and Evans, C.D.H. (2002) Assessment of guidelines for good practice in psychosocial care of mothers after stillbirth: a cohort study, *Lancet*, 360:9327, pp. 114–18.

Hurme, H. (1991) Dimensions of the grandparent role in Finland, in Smith, P.K. (ed.), *The Psychology of Grandparenthood: An International Perspective*. London: Routledge.

Iles, S. (1989) The loss of early pregnancy, Ch. 5 in Oates, M.R. (ed.), *Psychological Aspects of Obstetrics and Gynaecology*. London: Bailliere.

Illich, I. (1976) *Medical Nemesis: The Expropriation of Health*. New York: Pantheon Books.

James, N. (1992) Care = organization + physical labor + emotional labor, *Sociology of Health and Illness*, 14:4, pp. 488–509.

Jolly, J. (1987) *Missed Beginnings*, Croydon: Lisa Sainsbury Foundation/Austin Cornish.

Jones, A. (1989) Managing the invisible grief, *Senior Nurse*, May, 9:5, pp. 26–7.

Joseph, S. and Bailham, D. (2004) Traumatic childbirth: what we know and what we can do, *Midwives*, 7:6, pp. 258–61.

Jowett, S. (2003) Comments on 'occupational stress in nursing', *International Journal of Nursing Studies*, 40:5, pp. 567–9.

Kalish, R.A. (1985) *Death, Grief and Caring Relationships*, 2nd edn. Pacific Grove, Calif: Brooks Cole.

Kargar, I. (1990) Special pregnancies, *Community Outlook*, June, pp. 12–18.

Kastenbaum, R. (2000) *The Psychology of Death*. New York: Springer.

Katbamna, S. (2000) *'Race' and Childbirth*. Buckingham: Open University Press.

Kato, P.M. and Mann, T. (1999) A synthesis of psychological interventions for the bereaved, *Clinical Psychology Review*, 19:3, pp. 275–96.

Kaunonen, M., Tarkka, M., Paunonen, M. and Laippala, P. (1999) Grief and social support after the death of a spouse, *Journal of Advanced Nursing*, 30:6, pp. 1304–11.

Kaye, A.S. (1994) An interview with Kenneth Pike, *Current Anthropology*, 35:3, pp. 291–8.

Keleher, A.J., Theriault, R.L., Gwyn, K.M., Hunt, K.K. Stelling, C.B., Singletary, S.E., Ames, F.C., Buchholz, T.A., Sahin, A.A. and Kuerer, H.M. (2002) Multidisciplinary management of breast cancer concurrent with pregnancy, *Journal of the American College of Surgeons*, 194:1, pp. 54–64.

Kennell, J.H. and Klaus, M.H. (1982) Caring for the parents of premature or sick infants, in Klaus, M.H. and Kennell, J.H., *Parent–Infant Bonding*, 2nd edn. St Louis, Mo.: Mosby.

Kennell, J.H., Slyter, H. and Klaus, M.H. (1970) The mourning response of parents to the death of a newborn infant, *New England Journal of Medicine*, 283:7, pp. 344–9.

Kickbusch, I. (1989) Self-care in health promotion, *Social Science and Medicine*, 29:2, pp. 125–30.

Kirkham, M. (1999) The culture of midwifery in the National Health Service in England, *Journal of Advanced Nursing*, 30:3, pp. 732–9.

Kirkman, M. (2001) Thinking of something to say: public and private narratives of infertility, *Health Care for Women International*, 22:6, pp. 523–35.

Kirstjanson, L.J, McPhee, I., Pickstock, S., Wilson, D., Oldham, L. and Martin, K. (2001) Palliative care: nurses' perceptions of good and bad deaths and care expectations: a qualitative analysis, *International Journal of Palliative Nursing*, 7:3, pp. 129–39.

Klass, D. (1997) The deceased child in the psychic and social worlds of bereaved parents during the resolution of grief, *Death Studies*, 21:2, pp. 147–75.

Klaus, M.H. and Kennell, J.H. (1976) *Maternal–Infant Bonding: The Impact of Early Separation or Loss on Family Development*. St Louis, Mo.: Mosby.

Klaus, M.H. and Kennell, J.H. (1982) *Parent Infant Bonding*, 2nd edn. St Louis, Mo.: Mosby.

Koblinsky, M. and Campbell, O. (1999) id21 insights, Issue 32, http://www.id21.org/insights/insights32/insights-iss32-art06.html. Accessed 4 January 2005.

Kohner, N. (2000) Pregnancy loss and the death of a baby: parents' choices, Ch. 57, p. 355, in Dickenson, D., Johnson, M. and Katz, J.S. (eds), *Death, Dying and Bereavement*, 2nd edn. London: Open University Press/Sage.

Kohner, N. (2002) Evidence-based practice in the care and support of parents after the death of a baby: some comments on recent research, *MIDIRS Midwifery Digest*, 12:4, pp. 547–50.

Kohner, N. and Henley, A. (1992) *When a Baby Dies: The Experience of Late Miscarriage, Stillbirth and Neonatal Death.* London: SANDS/Pandora.

Kowalski, K.M. (1987) Perinatal loss and bereavement, in Sonstegard, L., Kowalski, K.M. and Jennings, B., *Women's Health: Crisis and Illness in Childbearing.* Orlando, Fla.: Grune & Stratton.

Kübler-Ross, E. (1970) *On Death and Dying.* London: Tavistock Publications.

Kunyk, D. and Olson, J.K. (2001) Clarification of conceptualizations of empathy, *Journal of Advanced Nursing*, 35:3, pp. 317–25.

Laakso, H. and Paunonen-Ilmonen, M. (2002) Mothers' experience of social support following the death of a child, *Journal of Clinical Nursing*, 11:2, pp. 176–85.

Lady, Jane Crewe Monument, http://www. artandarchitecture. org.uk/images/conway/cae2948e.html. Accessed 31 December 2004.

Larkin, K.R. (1990) Cancer and pregnancy, *NAACOGS Clinical Issues in Perinatal and Women's Health Nursing*, 1:2, pp. 255–61.

Lavender, T. and Walkinshaw, S.A. (1998) Can midwives reduce postpartum psychological morbidity? A randomised trial, *Birth*, 25:4, pp. 215–19.

Layne, L.L. (1999) *Transformative Motherhood: On Giving and Getting in a Consumer Culture.* New York/London: New York University Press.

Layne, L.L. (2003) Unhappy endings: a feminist reappraisal of the women's health movement from the vantage of pregnancy loss, *Social Science and Medicine*, 56:9, pp. 1881–91.

Lazarus, R. (1976) *Patterns of Adjustment.* New York: McGraw-Hill.

Lendrum, S. and Syme, G. (1992) *Gift of Tears: A Practical Approach to Loss and Bereavement Counselling.* London: Tavistock/Routledge.

Leon, I.G. (1990) *When a Baby Dies: Psychotherapy for Pregnancy and Newborn Loss.* New Haven, Conn: Yale University Press.

Leon, I.G. (1992) Commentary: providing versus packaging support for bereaved parents after perinatal loss, *Birth*, June, 19:2, pp. 89–91.

Lerum, C.W. and Lobiondo-Wood, G. (1989) The relationship of maternal age, quickening and physical symptoms of pregnancy to the development of maternal–fetal attachment, *Birth*, 16:1, pp. 13–17.

Lesser, J., Oakes, R. and Koniak-Griffin, D. (2003) Vulnerable adolescent mothers' perceptions of maternal role and HIV risk, *Health Care for Women International*, 24:6, pp. 513–28.

Lewis, E. (1976) The management of stillbirth: coping with an unreality, *Lancet*, 18 September, pp. 619–20.

Lewis, E. (1979a) Mourning by the family after a stillbirth or neonatal death, *Archives of Disease in Childhood*, 54, pp. 303–6.

Lewis, E. (1979b) Inhibition of mourning by pregnancy: psychopathology and management, British Medical Journal, 7 July, pp. 27–8.

Lewis, E. and Page, A. (1978) Failure to mourn a stillbirth, *British Journal of Medical Psychology*, 51, pp. 237–41.

Lewis, E. and Bourne, S. (1989) Perinatal death, in Oates, M. (ed.), *Psychological Aspects of Obstetrics and Gynaecology.* London: Bailliere Tindall.

Lewis, G. and Drife, J. (2004) *Confidential Enquiry into Maternal and Child Health. Why Mothers Die 2000–2002 Executive Summary and Key Findings*, 6th Report. London: Royal College of Obstetricians and Gynaecologists.

Lewis, G., Drife, J. and de Swiet, M. (2001) *Why Mothers Die 1997–99: Confidential Enquiries into Maternal Deaths.* London: National Institute for Clinical Excellence.

Lewis, H. (1978) Nothing was said sympathy-wise, *Social Work Today*, 110:45, p. 2479.

Lieberman, M.A. (1979) Analyzing change mechanisms in groups, in Lieberman, M.A., Borman L.D. *et al.*, *Self-Help Groups for Coping with Crisis*. San Francisco, Calif.: Jossey Bass.

Lin, S.X. and Lasker, J.N. (1996) Patterns of grief reaction after pregnancy loss, *American Journal of Orthopsychiatry*, 66:2, pp. 262–71.

Lindemann, E. (1944) Symptomatology and management of acute grief, *American Journal of Psychiatry*, 101, pp. 141–9.

Littlewood, J. (1992) *Aspects of Grief: Bereavement in Adult Life*. London: Tavistock/Routledge.

Long, J. (1992) Grief and loss in childbirth, *Midwives Chronicle*, March, 105:1250, pp. 51–4.

Loudon, I. (1992) *Death in Childbirth: An International Study of Maternal Care and Maternal Mortality 1800–1950*. Oxford: Clarendon Press.

Lovell, A. (1983) Women's reactions to late miscarriage, stillbirth and perinatal death, *Health Visitor*, September, 56, pp. 325–7.

Lovell, A. (1984) A bereavement with a difference: a study of late miscarriage, stillbirth and perinatal death. Polytechnic of the South Bank Sociology Department, Occasional Paper 4.

Lovell, A. (1997) Death at the beginning of life, Ch. 2, p. 29, in Field, D., Hockey, H. and Small, N. (eds), *Death, Gender and Ethnicity*, London: Routledge.

Lovell, H., Bokoula, C., Misra, S. and Speight, N. (1986) Mothers' reactions to perinatal death, *Nursing Times*, 12 November, 82:46, pp. 40–2.

Lugton, J. (1989) *Communicating with Dying People and their Relatives*. Croydon: Austen Cornish/Lisa Sainsbury Foundation.

Lumley, J. (1990) Through a glass darkly: ultrasound and prenatal bonding, *Birth*, December, 17:4, pp. 214–17.

Lumley, L.J. (1979) The development of maternal fetal bonding in the first pregnancy, in Carena, L. and Zichella, L. (eds), *Emotion and Reproduction 5th International Congress of Psychosomatic Obsterics and Gynaecology*. London: Academic Press.

Lupton, D. and Fenwick, J. (2001) 'They've forgotten that I'm the mum': constructing and practising motherhood in special care nurseries, *Social Science and Medicine*, 53:8, pp. 1011–21.

Mccabe, A. (2002) My experience of post childbirth trauma, *AIMS Journal*, 14:1, pp. 15–16.

McCaffery, M. (1979) *Nursing Management of the Patient in Pain*. New York: Lippincott.

McCalman, C.L. (2003) Barriers and motivators for low-income Brazilian women in metropolitan Belo Horizonte: insights for AIDS prevention, *Health Care for Women International*, 24:6, pp. 565–85.

McCourt, C. and Pearce, A. (2000) Does continuity of carer matter to women from minority ethnic groups?, *Midwifery*, 16:2, pp. 145–54.

McCreight, B.S. (2004) A grief ignored: narratives of pregnancy loss from a male perspective, *Sociology of Health and Illness*, 26:3, pp. 326–50.

McHaffie, H.E. (1991) A study of support for families with a VLBW baby. University of Edinburgh Nursing Research Unit.

McHaffie, H.E. (1992) Social support in the NNICU, *Journal of Advanced Nursing*, 17, pp. 279–87.

McHaffie, H.E. (2001) *Crucial Decisions at the Beginning of Life: Parents' Experiences of Treatment Withdrawal from Infants*. Abingdon: Radcliffe Medical.

McHaffie, H.E., Laing, I.A., Parker, M. and McMillan, J. (2001) Deciding for imperilled newborns: medical authority or parental autonomy?, *Journal of Medical Ethics*, 27:2, pp. 104–9.

Macleod, J. (1993) *An Introduction to Counselling*. Buckingham: Open University Press.

McNeil, J.N. (1986) Communicating with surviving children, in Rando, T. (ed.) *Parental Loss of a Child*, Champaign, Ill.: Research Press.

Macrory, F. (2003) HIV and maternal health: the Manchester response, *MIDIRS Midwifery Digest*, 13:1, pp. 51–3.

Maine, D. and Rosenfield, A. (1999) The Safe Motherhood Initiative: why has it stalled?, *American Journal of Public Health*, 89:4, pp. 480–2.

Mallinson, G. (1989) Life crises: when a baby dies, *Nursing Times*, 1 March, 85:9, pp. 31–4.

Mandell, F. and Wolfe, L.C. (1975) Sudden Infant Death Syndrome and subsequent pregnancy, *Pediatrics*, 56:5, pp. 774–6.

Mander, R. (1992a) The control of pain in labour, *Journal of Clinical Nursing*, 1:4, pp. 219–23.

Mander, R. (1992b) See how they learn: experience as the basis of practice, *Nurse Education Today*, February 12:1, pp. 11–18.

Mander, R. (1992c) Seeking approval for research access: the gatekeepers' role in facilitating a study of the care of the relinquishing mother, *Journal of Advanced Nursing*, December, 17:12, pp. 1460–4.

Mander, R. (1992d) *Research Report: Midwives' Care of the Relinquishing Mother*. London: Iolanthe Trust.

Mander, R. (1995a) Midwife researchers need to get their work published, *British Journal of Midwifery*, 3:2, pp. 107–10.

Mander, R. (1995b) *The Care of the Mother Grieving a Baby Relinquished for Adoption*. Aldershot: Avebury.

Mander, R. (1996) The grieving mother: care in the community?, *Modern Midwife*, 6:8, pp. 10–13.

Mander, R. (1999a) The significance of hierarchy in a research project on adoption and adaptation, *Midwifery*, 15:2, pp. 129–38.

Mander, R. (1999b) The death of a mother – a proposed research project, *RCM Midwives Journal*, 2:1, pp. 24–5.

Mander, R. (1999c) Preliminary report: a study of the midwife's experience of the death of a mother, *RCM Midwives Journal*, 2:11, pp. 346–9.

Mander, R. (2000) Perinatal grief: understanding the bereaved and their carers, Ch. 3, pp. 29–50, in Alexander, J., Levy, V. and Roth, C. (eds), *Midwifery Practice: Core Topics* 3. London: Macmillan.

Mander, R. (2001a) Death of a mother: taboo and the midwife, *Practising Midwife*, 4:8, pp. 23–5.

Mander, R. (2001b) The midwife's ultimate paradox: a UK-based study of the death of a mother, *Midwifery*, 17:4, pp. 248–59.

Mander, R. (2001c) *Supportive Care and Midwifery*. Oxford: Blackwell Science.

Mander, R. (2004a) *Men and Maternity*. London: Routledge.

Mander, R. (2004b) When the professional gets personal – the midwife's experience of the death of a mother, *Evidence Based Midwifery*, 2:2, pp. 40–5.

Mander, R. and Haroldsdottir, E. (2002) Palliative care and childbearing, *European Journal of Palliative Care*, 9:6, pp. 240–2.

Mander, R. and Marshall, R.K. (2003) An historical analysis of the role of paintings and photographs in comforting bereaved parents, *Midwifery*, 19:3, pp. 230–42.

Marck, P.B. (1994) Unexpected pregnancy: the uncharted land of women's experience, Ch. 3, pp. 82–138, in Field, P.A. and Marck, P.B. (eds), *Uncertain Motherhood: Negotiating the Risks of the Childbearing Years*. Thousand Oaks, Calif./London: Sage.

Marris, P. (1986) *Loss and Change*. London: Routledge and Kegan Paul.

Marshall, R.K. (1976) *Childhood in Seventeenth Century Scotland*. Edinburgh: Scottish National Portrait Gallery.

Marshall, R.K. (1983) *Virgins and Viragos: A History of Women in Scotland from 1080 to 1980*. London: Collins.

Marshall, R.K. (2004) Personal communication.

Martin, J. (2000) Doctor's mask on pain, in Dickenson, D., Johnson, M. and Katz, J.S. (eds), *Death, Dying and Bereavement*, 2nd edn. London: Open University Press/Sage.

Maslach, C. (1982) *Burnout: The Cost of Caring*. New York: Prentice Hall.

Menage, J. (1993) Post-traumatic stress disorder in women who have undergone obstetric and/or gynaecological procedures, *Journal of Reproductive and Infant Psychology*, 11:4, pp. 221–8.

Menning, B.E. (1982) The psychosocial impact of infertility, *Nursing Clinics of North America*, March, 17:1, pp. 155–63.

Menzies, I.E.P. (1969) The functioning of social systems as a defence against anxiety, in MacGuire, J. (ed.), *Threshold to Nursing*. London: Bell.

Metts, S., Geist, P. and Gray, J.L. (1994) The role of relationship characteristics in the provision and effectiveness of supportive messages among nursing professionals, Ch. 12, p. 229, in Burleson, B.R., Albrecht, T.L. and Sarason, I.G. (eds), *Communication of Social Support*. London: Sage.

Miller, E. and Webb, B. (1988) *The Nature of Effective Self-help Support in Different Contexts*. London: Tavistock Institute of Human Relations.

Monteith, R. (1704) An theatre of mortality; or, the illustrious inscriptions extant upon the several monuments ... within the Grayfriars church-yard; and other churches and burial-places within the city of Edinburgh and suburbs. Edinburgh.

Morrin, N. (1983) As great a loss, *Nursing Mirror*, 16 February, 156:7, p. 33.

Morse, J.M. (1989) Strategies for sampling, Ch. 8 in Morse, J.M. (ed.), *Qualitative Nursing Research: A Contemporary Dialogue*. London: Sage.

Moulder, C. (1998) *Understanding Pregnancy Loss: Perspectives and Issues in Care*. London: Macmillan.

Moyzakitis, W. (2004) Exploring women's descriptions of distress and/or trauma of childbirth from a feminist perspective, *RCM Evidence Based Midwifery*, 2:1, pp. 8–14.

Mpshe, W.S., Gmeiner, A. and van Wyk, S. (2002) Experiences of black adolescents who chose to terminate their pregnancies, *Health SA Gesondheid*, 7:1, pp. 68–81.

Munch, E. (1899–1900) *The Dead Mother*, Kunsthalle, Bremen, http://www.ibiblio.org/wm/paint/auth/munch/. Accessed 31 December 2004.

Munro, L., Rodwell, J. and Harding, L. (1998) Assessing occupational stress in psychiatric nurses using the full job strain model: the value of social support to nurses, *International Journal of Nursing Studies*, 35:6, pp. 339–45.

Murphy, F.A. (1998) The experience of early miscarriage from a male perspective, *Journal of Clinical Nursing*, 7:4, pp. 325–32.

Murphy-Black, T. (2000) Questionnaire, Ch. 23 in Cormack, D. (ed.), *The Research Process in Nursing*. Oxford: Blackwell Science.

Murray, J. and Callan, V.J. (1988) Predicting adjustment to perinatal death, *British Journal of Medical Psychology*, 61, pp. 237–44.

Mussen, P.H., Janeway, J., Kagan, J. and Huston, A.C. (1990) *Child Personality and Development*. New York: Harper & Row.

Newman, R.B. (1998) Obstetric management in high-order pregnancies, Ch. 8 in Neilson, J.P. (ed.), *Bailliere's Clinical Obstetrics and Gynaecology*, 12:1, Multiple Pregnancy, pp. 109–30.

NHS CRD (2001) *Counselling in Primary Care Effectiveness Matters*. NHS Centre for Reviews and Dissemination, www.york.ac.uk/inst/crd/pdf/em52.pdf. Accessed 20 August 2004.

Nichols, J.A. (1986) Newborn death, in Rando, T.A. (ed.), *Parental Loss of Child*. Champaign, Ill.: Research Press.

Nikcevic, A.V., Kuczmierczyk, A.R., Tunkel, S.A. and Nicolaides, K.H. (2000) Distress after miscarriage: relation to the knowledge of the cause of pregnancy loss and coping style, *Journal of Reproductive and Infant Psychology*, 18:4, pp. 339–43.

Niven, C.A. (1992) *Psychological Care for Families: Before, During and After Birth*. Oxford: Butterworth-Heinemann.

Nord, D. (1997) *Multiple AIDS-related Loss*. Washington, DC: Taylor & Francis.

Oakley, A., McPherson, A. and Roberts, H. (1990) *Miscarriage*. London: Penguin.

O'Connor, M., Nikoletti, S., Kristjanson, L.J., Loh, R. and Willcock, B. (2003) Writing therapy for the bereaved: evaluation of an intervention, *Journal of Palliative Medicine*, 6:2, pp. 195–204.

Oglethorpe, R.J.L. (1989) Parenting after perinatal bereavement: a review of the literature, *Journal of Reproductive and Infant Psychology*, 7:4, pp. 227–44.

O'Neill, B. and Fallon, M. (1997) Clinical review ABC of palliative care: principles of palliative care and pain control, *British Medical Journal*, 315, pp. 801–4.

Osterweis, M., Solomon, F. and Green, M. (1984) *Bereavement: Reactions: Consequences and Care*. Committee for the Study of the Health Consequences of the Stress of Bereavement. Washington, DC: National Academy Press.

Parkes, C.M. (1976) *Bereavement: Studies of Grief in Adult Life*. Harmondsworth: Penguin.

Parkes, C.M. (1980) Bereavement counselling: does it work?, *British Medical Journal*, 282:4, pp. 3–6.

Parkes, C.M. (1987) *Bereavement: Studies of Grief in Adult Life*, 2nd edn. London: Tavistock.

Parkes, C.M. (1996) *Bereavement: Studies of Grief in Adult Life*, 3rd edn. London: Tavistock.

Penson, J.M. (1990) *Bereavement: A Guide for Nurses*. London: Harper & Row.

Peppers, L.G. and Knapp, R.J. (1980) Maternal reactions to involuntary fetal/infant death, *Psychiatry*, 43, pp. 155–9.

Peppers, L. and Knapp, R. (1982) *Motherhood and Mourning*. New York: Praeger.

Pereira, H. (2004) The arrival of a rival, NHS Mother and Child, http://www.cyworks.co.uk/nhsmother/pdf/MAC2PDFs/thearrivaofarival.pdf. Accessed 27 July 2004.

Petterson, B., Blair, E., Watson, L. and Stanley, F. (1998) Adverse outcome after multiple pregnancy, Ch. 1 in Neilson, J.P. (ed.), *Bailliere's Clinical Obstetrics and Gynaecology*, 12:1, Multiple Pregnancy, pp. 1–18.

Phoenix, A. (1990) Black women and the maternity services, in Garcia, J., Kilpatrick, R. and Richards, M. (eds), *The Politics of Maternity Care: Services for Childbearing Women in Twentieth-Century Britain.* Oxford: Oxford University Press.

Pierucci, R.L., Kirby, R.S. and Leuthner, S.R. (2001) End-of-life care for neonates and infants: the experience and effects of a palliative care consultation service, *Pediatrics,* 108:3, pp. 653–60.

Pongruenphant, R. and Tyson, P.D. (2000) When nurses cry: coping with occupational stress in Thailand, *International Journal of Nursing Studies,* 37:6, pp. 535–9.

Porter, S. and Carter, D. (2000) Common terms and concepts in research, Ch. 2, pp. 17–28 in Cormack, D.F.S. (ed.), *The Research Process in Nursing,* 4th edn. Oxford: Blackwell Scientific.

Price, F. (1992) Having triplets, quads or quins; who bears the responsibility?, Ch. 5 in Stacey, M. (ed.), *Changing Human Reproduction: Social Science Perspectives.* London: Sage.

Priest, S. (2000) Viewpoint. Support when a baby dies, *RCM Midwives Journal,* 3:6, p. 185.

Primeau, M.R. and Lamb, J.M. (1995) When a baby dies: rights of the baby and parents, *Journal of Obstetric, Gynecologic, and Neonatal Nursing,* 24:3, pp. 206–8.

Puddifoot, J.E. and Johnson, M.P. (1997) The legitimacy of grieving: the partner's experience at miscarriage, *Social Science and Medicine,* 45:6, pp. 837–45.

Puddifoot, J.E. and Johnson, M.P. (1999) Active grief, despair, and difficulty coping: some measured characteristics of male response following their partner's miscarriage, *Journal of Reproductive and Infant Psychology,* 17:2, pp. 89–94.

Queenan, J. (1978) The ultimate defeat, *Contemporary Obstetrics and Gynaecology,* 11, p. 7.

Rådestad, I., Nordin, C., Steineck, G. and Sjogren, B. (1996a) Stillbirth is no longer managed as a nonevent: a nationwide study in Sweden, *Birth,* 23:4, pp. 209–15.

Rådestad, I., Steineck, G., Nordin, C. and Sjogren, B. (1996b) Psychological complications after stillbirth: influence of memories and immediate management: population based study, *British Medical Journal,* 312, pp. 1505–8.

Rådestad, I., Nordin, C., Steineck, G. and Sjogren, B. (1998) A comparison of women's memories of care during pregnancy, labour and delivery after stillbirth or live birth, *Midwifery,* 14:2, pp. 111–17.

Rajan, L. (1994) Social isolation and support in pregnancy loss, *Health Visitor,* 67:3, pp. 97–101.

Rajan, L. and Oakley, A. (1993) No pills for the heartache: the importance of social support for women who suffer pregnancy loss, *Journal of Reproductive and Infant Psychology,* 11:2, pp. 75–88.

Rankin, J., Wright, C. and Lind, T. (2002) Cross sectional survey of parents' experience and views of the post-mortem examination, *British Medical Journal,* 324, pp. 816–18.

Raphael, B. (1982) The young child and the death of a parent, in Parkes, C.M. and Stevenson-Hinde, J. (eds), *The Place of Attachment in Human Behaviour.* New York: Basic Books.

Raphael, B. (1984) *The Anatomy of Bereavement: A Handbook for the Caring Professions.* London: Unwin Hyman.

Raphael-Leff, J. (1991) *Psychological Processes of Childbearing.* London: Chapman & Hall.

Raphael-Leff, J. (1993) *Pregnancy: The Inside Story.* London: Sheldon.

Reading, A.E. (1989) The measurement of fetal attachment over the course of pregnancy, in van Hall, E.V. and Everaerd, W. (eds), *The Free Woman: Women's Health in the 1990s*. Carnforth: Parthenon.

Redman, C. (2003) Psychological issues. Counselling in perinatal loss, *British Journal of Midwifery*, 11:12, pp. 731–4.

Redshaw, M.E., Harris, A. and Ingram, J.C. (1996) *Delivering Neonatal Care: The Neonatal Unit as a Working Environment; A Survey of Neonatal Unit Nursing*. London: HMSO.

Reid, M. (1990) Prenatal diagnosis and screening, Ch. 16 in Garcia, J., Kilpatrick, R. and Richards, M. (eds), *The Politics of Maternity Care: Services for Childbearing Women in Twentieth-Century Britain*. Oxford: Oxford University Press.

Reyes Frausto, S., Bobadilla Fernandez, J.L., Karchmer Krivitzky, S. and Martinez Gonzalez, L. (1998) Effect of maternal death on family dynamics and infant survival, *Ginecologia y Obstetricia de Mexico*, 66, pp. 428–33.

Reynolds, S. (1997) Psychological well-being at work: is prevention better than cure?, *Journal of Psychosomatic Research*, 43: 1, pp. 93–102.

Richards, M.P.M. (1983) Parent–child relationships: some general considerations, in Davis, J.A., Richards, M.P.M. and Roberton, N.R.C., *Parent–Baby Attachment in Premature Infants*. London: Croom Helm.

Richards, M.P.M. (1989) Social and ethical problems of fetal diagnosis and screening, *Journal of Reproductive and Infant Psychology*, 7:2, pp. 171–85.

Richards, M.P.M. and Hawthorne, J.T. (1999) Psychological aspects of neonatal care, Ch. 5, pp. 61–72, in Rennie, J.M. and Roberton, N.R.C. (eds), *A Manual of Neonatal Intensive Care*, 4th edn. London: Arnold.

Richardson, A. and Goodman, M. (1983) *Self-help and Social Care: Mutual Aid Organisations in Practice*. London: Policy Studies Institute.

Rillstone, P. and Hutchinson, S.A. (2001) Managing the reemergence of anguish: pregnancy after a loss due to anomalies, *Journal of Obstetric, Gynecologic, and Neonatal Nursing*, 30:3, pp. 291–8.

Robak, R.W. (1999) Loss, death, bereavement: where are the empirical studies?, *Psychological Reports*, 84:2, pp. 701–2.

Robb, F. (1999) Professional issues. Congenital malformations: breaking the bad news, *British Journal of Midwifery*, 7:1, pp. 26–31.

Roberts, K.S. (2003) The long road home. Providing culturally sensitive care to the childbearing Islamic family, part II, *Advances in Neonatal Care*, 3:5, pp. 250–5.

Robinson, L. and Mahon, M.M. (1997) Sibling bereavement: a concept analysis, *Death Studies*, 21:5, pp. 477–99.

Roch, S. (1987) Sharing the grief, *Nursing Times*, 8 April, 83:14, pp. 52–3.

Rose, S., Bisson, J. and Wessely, S. (2003) Psychological debriefing for preventing post traumatic stress disorder (PTSD) (Cochrane Review), in *The Cochrane Library*, Issue 4. Chichester, UK: John Wiley.

Rose, X. (1990) *Widow's Journey: A Return to Living*. London: Souvenir Press.

Rothman, B.K. (1986) *The Tentative Pregnancy: Prenatal Diagnosis and the Future of Motherhood*. London: Pandora.

Rothman, B.K. (1990) Commentary: women feel social and economic pressures to abort abnormal fetuses, *Birth*, 17:2, p. 81.

Rowe, J., Clyman, R., Green, C., Mikkelson, C., Haight, J. and Ataide, L. (1978) Follow-up of families who experienced a perinatal death, *Pediatrics*, 62:2, pp. 166–9.

Rowsell, E., Jongman, G., Kilby, M., Kirchmeier, R. and Orford, J. (2001) The psychological impact of recurrent miscarriage, and the role of counselling at a pre-pregnancy counselling clinic, *Journal of Reproductive and Infant Psychology*, 19:1, pp. 33–45.

Rubin, R. (1967) Attachment of the maternal role, *Nursing Research*, 16:3, pp. 237–45.

Ruiz, L. (2001) Withholding developmental care: is it ethical?, *Journal of Neonatal Nursing*, 7:6, pp. 209–13.

Rynearson, E.K. (1982) Psychotherapy of pathologic grief: revisions and limitations, *Psychiatric Clinics of North America*, September, 10:3, pp. 487–99.

Säflund, K., Sjögren, B. and Wredling, R. (2004) The role of caregivers after a stillbirth: views and experiences of parents, *Birth*, 31:2, pp. 132–7.

Salladay, S. and Cavender, K. (1992) Post-abortion syndrome: dealing with guilt and grief, *Journal of Christian Nursing*, 9:2, pp. 18–21.

Samuelsson, M., Radestad, I. and Segesten, K. (2001) A waste of life: fathers' experience of losing a child before birth, *Birth* 28:2, pp. 124–30.

SANDS (1995) *Guidelines for Professionals: Pregnancy Loss and the Death of a Baby*, rev. edn. London: SANDS.

SANDS (2004) How to contact us, http://www.uk-sands.org/. Accessed 3 September 2004.

Sarason, I.G., Sarason, B.R. and Pierce, G.R. (1994) Relationship specific social support: towards a model for the analysis of supportive interactions, Ch. 5 p. 91, in Burleson, B.R., Albrecht, T.L. and Sarason, I.G. (eds), *Communication of Social Support*. London: Sage.

Schofield, R. (1986) Did the mother really die? Three centuries of maternal mortality in 'The world we have lost', Ch. 9, p. 231, in Bonfield, L., Smith, R.M. and Wrightson, K. (eds), *The World We Have Gained: Histories of Population and Social Structure*. Oxford: Blackwell.

SEHD (2004) *Nursing for Health: The Effectiveness of Public Health Nursing: A Review of Systematic Reviews*, http://www.scotland.gov.uk/library3/health/ephn/ephn-26.asp. Accessed 20 August 2004.

Selye, H. (1956) *The Stress of Life*. New York: McGraw-Hill.

Selye, H. (1980) Stress and a holistic view of health for the nursing profession, in Claus, K. and Bailey, J. (eds), *Living with Stress and Promoting Well-being*. St Louis, Mo.: Mosby.

Sherr, L. (1989) Death of a baby, in Sherr, L., *Death, Dying and Bereavement*, London: Blackwell Scientific.

Sherr, L. (1995a) *Grief and AIDS*. Chichester: Wiley.

Sherr, L. (1995b) Book review, *Child Care, Health and Development*, 21:6.

Sherratt, D. (1987) What do you say?, *Midwives Chronicle*, August, 100:1195, pp. 235–6.

Shiffman, J. (2003) Generating political will for safe motherhood in Indonesia, *Social Science and Medicine*, 56:6, pp. 1197–207.

Silverman, P.R. and Klass, D. (1996) Introduction: What's the problem?, Ch. 1, p. 3, in Klass, D., Silverman, P.R. and Nickman, S.L. (eds), *Continuing Bonds: New Understandings of Grief*. Washington, DC: Taylor & Francis.

Simmons, M. (1992) Helping children grieve, *Nursing Times*, 9 December, 88:50, pp. 30–2.

Simonds, W. (2002) Watching the clock: keeping time during pregnancy, birth, and postpartum experiences, *Social Science and Medicine*, 55:4, pp. 559–70.

Singg, S. (2003) Parents and the death of a child, in Bryant, C.D. (ed.), *Handbook of Death and Dying*, Vol. 2, Part VII, pp. 880–8. Thousand Oaks, Calif.: Sage.

Small, R., Lumley, J., Donohue, L., Potter, A. and Waldenström, U. (2000) Randomised controlled trial of midwife led debriefing to reduce maternal depression after operative childbirth, *British Medical Journal*, 321, pp. 1043–7.

Smith, M.S. (1991) An evolutionary perspective on grandparent–grandchild relationships, in Smith, P.K. (ed.), *The Psychology of Grandparenthood: An International Perspective*. London: Routledge.

Smith, R. (2003) Death, come closer, *British Medical Journal*, 327:7408, p. 173.

Solnit, A.J. and Stark, M.H. (1961) Mourning and the birth of a defective child, *Psychoanalytic Study of the Child*, 16:1, pp. 523–37.

Sorosky, A.D., Baran, A. and Pannor, R. (1984) *The Adoption Triangle*. New York: Anchor.

SPCERH (2003) *The Scottish Audit of the Management of Early Pregnancy Loss*, http://www.show.scot.nhs.uk/spcerh/.

Stack, J. (1982) *Reproductive Casualties*. New York: Perinatal Press.

Stainton, M.C. (1990) Parents' awareness of their unborn infant in the third trimester, *Birth*, June, 17:2, pp. 92–6.

Stapleton, H., Duerden, J. and Kirkham, M. (1998) *Evaluation of the Impact of the Supervision of Midwives on Professional Practice and the Quality of Midwifery Care*. Sheffield/London: University of Sheffield and English National Board for Nursing Midwifery and Health Visiting.

Statham, H. and Dimavicius, J. (1992) Commentary: how do you give the bad news to parents, *Birth*, 19:2, pp. 103–4.

Steele, A.M. and Beadle, M. (2003) A survey of postnatal debriefing, *Journal of Advanced Nursing*, 43:2, pp. 130–6.

Stephenson, N. and Corben, V. (1997) Phenomenology, Ch. 5, pp. 115–38, in Smith, P. (ed.), *Research Mindedness for Practice*. Edinburgh: Churchill Livingstone.

Stone, L. (1977) *The Family, Sex and Marriage in England, 1500–1800*. London: Weidenfeld & Nicolson.

Stray-Pedersen, B. and Stray-Pedersen, S. (1984) Etiologic factors and subsequent reproductive performance in 195 couples with a prior history of habitual abortion, *American Journal of Obstetrics and Gynaecology*, 148:2, pp. 140–6.

Stroebe, M. and Schut, H. (1995) The dual process model of coping with bereavement: rationale and description, *Death Studies*, 23:3, pp. 197–224.

Stroebe, W. and Stroebe, M.S. (1987) *Bereavement and Health: The Psychological and Physical Consequences of Partner Loss*. Cambridge: Cambridge University Press.

Swanson, K.M. (1999) Clinical scholarship: research-based practice with women who have had miscarriages, *Image – the Journal of Nursing Scholarship*, 31:4, pp. 339–45.

Swanson, K.M., Karmali, Z.A., Powell, S.H. and Pulvermakher, F. (2003) Miscarriage effects on couples' interpersonal and sexual relationships during the first year after loss: women's perceptions, *Psychosomatic Medicine*, 65:5, pp. 902–10.

Swanson, P.B., Pearsall-Jones, J.G. and Hay, D.A. (2002) How mothers cope with the death of a twin or higher multiple, *Twin Research*, 5:3, pp. 156–64.

Symington, A. and Pinelli, J. (2004) Developmental care for promoting development and preventing morbidity in preterm infants (Cochrane Review), in *The Cochrane Library*, Issue 3. Chichester, UK: John Wiley.

TCF (2002) The Compassionate Friends, http://www.compassionatefriends.org/survey.shtml. Accessed 27 July 2004.

TCF (2003) When your grandchild dies. The Compassionate Friends, http://www.tcf.org.uk/leaflets/legrandchildren.html. Accessed 27 July 2004.

Tentoni, S.C. (1995) A therapeutic approach to reduce postabortion grief in university women, *Journal of American College Health*, 44:1, pp. 35–7.

Thompson, A. (1999) Poor and pregnant in Africa: safe motherhood and human rights, *Midwifery*, 15:3, pp. 146–53.

Thompson, A. (2003) Safe motherhood at risk?, *Midwifery*, 12:4, pp. 159–64.

Thompson, N. (1997) Masculinity and loss, Ch. 4 in Field, D., Hockey, J. and Small, N. (eds), *Death, Gender and Ethnicity*, London: Routledge.

Thomson, A. (1999) Remember maternal mortality, *Midwifery*, 15:3, p. 145.

Thomson, A. (2003) The relationship of the legalisation of midwifery and safe motherhood, *Midwifery*, 19:2, pp. 77–8.

Thoresen, L. (2003) A reflection on Cicely Saunders' views on a good death through the philosophy of Charles Taylor, *International Journal of Palliative Nursing*, 9:1, pp. 19–23.

Tschudin, V. (1997) *Counselling for Loss and Bereavement*. London: Baillière Tindall.

Turrill, S. (1992) Supported positioning in intensive care, *Paediatric Nursing*, May, 4:4, pp. 24–7.

Turton, P., Hughes, P., Evans, C.D. and Fainman, D. (2001) Incidence, correlates and predictors of post-traumatic stress disorder in the pregnancy after stillbirth, *British Journal of Psychiatry*, 178, pp. 556–60.

Vance, J.C., Boyle, F.M., Najman, J.M. and Thearle, M.J. (2002) Couple distress after sudden infant or perinatal death: a 30 month follow up, *Journal of Paediatrics and Child Health*, 38:4, pp. 368–72.

Van Wyk, B., Pillay, V., Swartz, L. and Zwarenstein, M. (2004) Preventive staff-support interventions for health workers (Protocol for a Cochrane Review), in *The Cochrane Library*, Issue 3. Chichester, UK: John Wiley.

Vera, M.I. (2003) Social dimensions of grief, in Bryant, C.D. (ed.), *Handbook of Death and Dying*, Part VI, pp. 838–46. Thousand Oaks, Calif.: Sage.

Videka-Sherman, L.M. (1982) Coping with the death of a child, *American Journal of Orthopsychiatry*, 51:4, pp. 699–703.

Vogel, H.P. and Knox, E.G. (1975) Reproductive patterns after stillbirth and early infant death, *Journal of Biosocial Science*, 7, pp. 103–11.

Wagner, R.E., Hexel, M., Bauer, W.W. and Kropiunigg, U. (1997) Crying in hospitals: a survey of doctors', nurses' and medical students' experience and attitudes, *Medical Journal of Australia*, 166:1, pp. 13–16.

Walker, R. (1992) One from the heart, *Nursing Times*, 88:1, p. 27.

Walter, E.B., Royce, R.A., Fernandez, M.I., Dehovitz, J., Ickovics, J.R. and Lampe, M.A. (2001) Perinatal Guidelines Evaluation Project group. New mothers' knowledge and attitudes about perinatal human immunodeficiency virus infection, *Obstetrics and Gynecology*, 97:1, pp. 70–6.

Walter, T. (1999) *On Bereavement: The Culture of Grief*. Philadelphia, Penn.: Open University Press.

Walter, T. (2003) Historical and cultural variants on the good death, *British Medical Journal*, 327:7408, pp. 218–20.

Watson, N. (1993) Personal communication.

Werner, N.P. and Conway, A.E. (1990) Caregiver contacts experinced by premature infants in a NNICU, *Maternal–Child Nursing Journal*, Spring, 19:1, pp. 21–43.

Weston, R., Martin, T. and Anderson, Y. (1998) *Loss and Bereavement: Managing Change*. Oxford: Blackwell Scientific.

White, W.L. (2004) Addiction recovery mutual aid groups: an enduring international phenomenon, *Addiction*, 99:5, pp. 532–8.

Wilson, J. (1995) *Two Worlds: Self Help Groups and Professionals*. Birmingham: British Association of Social Workers.

Wolff, J.R., Nielson, P.E. and Schiller, P. (1970) The emotional reaction to stillbirth, *American Journal of Obstetrics and Gynaecology*, 108:1, pp. 73–7.

Wolke, D. (1987a) Environmental and developmental neonatology, *Journal of Reproductive and Infant Psychology*, 5:1, pp. 17–42.

Wolke, D. (1987b) Environmental neonatology, *Archives of Disease in Childhood*, October, 62:10, pp. 987–8.

Wood, D. (1998) *How Children Think and Learn*, 2nd edn. Oxford: Blackwell.

Woodger, J. (2000) Professional issues. Adoption: how to support the relinquishing mother, *British Journal of Midwifery*, 8:1, pp. 9–12.

Woodward, S., Pope, A., Robson, W.J. and Hagan, O. (1985) Bereavement counselling after sudden death, *British Medical Journal*, February, 290:2, pp. 363–5.

Woollett, A. and Dosanjh-Matwala, N. (1990) Postnatal care: the attitudes and experiences of Asian women in east London, *Midwifery*, 6:4, pp. 178–84.

Worden, J.W. (2003) *Grief Counselling and Grief Therapy: A Handbook for the Mental Health Practitioner*, 3rd edn. New York: Brunner-Routledge.

World Health Organisation (WHO) (1983) *Self-help and Health in Europe*. Copenhagen: World Health Organisation Regional Office for Europe.

World Health Organisation (WHO) (2004) *Maternal Mortality in 2000: Estimates Developed by WHO, UNICEF, UNFPA*. Geneva: WHO.

Wright, K.B. and Bell, S.B. (2003) Health-related support groups on the internet: linking empirical findings to social support and computer-mediated communication theory, *Journal of Health Psychology*, 8:1, pp. 39–54.

Yates, D.W., Ellison, G. and McGuiness, S. (1993) Care of the suddenly bereaved, in Dickenson, D. and Johnson, M. (eds), *Death, Dying and Bereavement*, London: Open University Press/Sage.

Yeats, W.B. (1899) He wishes for the cloths of heaven, from Yeats, W.B. (1933) *The Collected Poems of W.B. Yeats*. London: Macmillan.

Young, N. and Bennett, R. (2002) Visiting women after a termination, *British Journal of Midwifery*, 10:1, pp. 30–4.

Zimmermann, C. and Rodin, G. (2004) The denial of death thesis: sociological critique and implications for palliative care, *Palliative Medicine*, March, 18:2, pp. 121–8.

Zorlu, C.G., Yalcin, H.R., Caglar, T. and Gokmen, O. (1997) Conservative management of twin pregnancies with one dead fetus: is it safe?, *Acta Obstetricia et Gynecologica Scandinavica*, 76:2, pp. 128–30.

Index

acceptance xii, 83
accident and emergency department 85
accommodation 75
actualising the loss 83
advance directive 120
AIDS orphans 100
aims of care 59
alleviating stress 156
anger 71, 123; unfocussed 87, 152
anniversaries 73
anniversary baby 201, 204
anticipatory grieving 38, 113
approach to care 58
assumptions 209
asymmetry 97
attachment 7, 13, 202
awareness 91

baby 4; as individual 68
bad news 59
balance of power 188
behaviour 2
behaviourism 13
being available 73
being caught in a trap 182
being in a crisis 184
being strong 93
bereavement 3; counselling 79;
    specialist 59; team 32
biography 8, 192
birth: experience of 18; as good
    experience 69
blame 94, 95
blaming survivor 102
bonding 15, 24
Bourne, S. 11, 145
Bowlby, J. 7, 14, 21
breaking bad news 46, 117, 94
breastfeeding 57

burial 210
burnout 156

care after the decision to discontinue
    treatment 124
caution 183
changing attitudes 126
checklist 58
choices and control 75
chronic niceness 162
client 82
client-centredness 84
closed circle 158
'cock-ups' 24, 62
Cocoanut Grove incident 21
cognitive-behavioural counselling 82
collegial support 157
comfort and medical care 120
communication 90, 95, 105, 116;
    between parents 118; with staff 61;
    with woman 61
community 24, 32, 87
Compassionate Friends, The (TCF) 187,
    194
complexity of emotional processes 36
concentrated support 203
conception plans 198
concerns 110
confidence building 184
confirming who died 34
conflicted grief 11
congruence 83
conspiracy of silence 36, 91, 138
consumerist ethos 180
contact 27; with baby 63; decision to
    63; encouraging 63; establishing 181
continuing support 83
contrasting the mother's own earlier
    expectations 37

control 74, 173
conversations 34
coping mechanism 94, 121, 170
cot 65
counselling process 82
counsellor 84
couple differences 92, 96
creating memories 67
creativity 207
critical incident technique 167
critical reading 21
criticisms of care 24
crying real tears 171
cultural assumptions 60
cultural implications 43
culture 2, 60, 143, 208

danger of childbirth 130
death day 204
deciding initiating/continuing treatment 122
decision-making 45
definitions 2
denial 9, 39, 75
dependent grief 11
depression 64
design 25
developing awareness 9
developing countries 143
developmental growth 1
developmental stage 103
different grieving 197
difficulty 149
disapproving 169
disaster 139
disbelief 110
discontinuity of care 155
dissynchrony 97
distance 170
dogma 26
double bind 96
drop out rate 22
dual process 7, 96
duration of grief 199
duration of hospital stay 76

educating 87
effect of pregnancy on grief 200
effectiveness 81
emic approach 28
emotion work 165
emotional labour 165
emotional support 36
empathy 83

empowerment 180
encouragement 157
encouraging acknowledgement 87
environment 126
ethical implications 80
ethics 93
ethnic minority groups 33
evaluation 80, 194
evaluative research 179
evidence-base 194
expectations 91
experiment 22
experts xi

facilitating communication 118
factors making grief less difficult 111
factors making grief more difficult 112
failure 146; to mourn 199
family xii, 23, 71, 89; disintegration of 134; and maternal death 134; support 73
fantasy baby 18
father 34, 92, 193
fathoming complexity 71
feedback 190
fertility rate 201
fetus 4
field notes 30
focus for grief 35
Forrest, G.C. 80
funeral 72; service 163
future childbearing 73
future pregnancy 196

gatekeepers 27
general adaptation syndrome 'gas' 148
gestalt 89
gestation/age 23
giving information 87
Gohlish, C. 5, 76
good death 6
Gorer, G. 1
grandparents 99, 134
gratitude 101
grief 2; therapy 79; work 6
grieving one 102
group cohesion 138; counselling 163
guilt 9, 40, 61, 100, 104

have another 196
Hawthorne effect 26, 80
helper-therapy principle 179
helping the carers 190
hidden meanings 197

historical death 130
HIV testing 56
home visits by the midwife 77
homeostasis 89, 90
honesty and directness 59
hospital visiting 32
hospital-based support groups 188
human contact 80
hyperidealisation 204

identifying and expressing 83
identifying defences and coping
    mechanisms 83
identifying pathology 83
ignorance of existence 184
implications for professionals 188
imprinting 13
inability to cry 176
inability to help 100
inadequacy 153
inducing labour 38
infertility 53
information 190
information-giving 116
initiating treatment 122
inside baby 18
interactionist stress 148
interdisciplinary support group 161
international death rate 133
internet 179; self-help on 190
interventions 160
intimacy of loss 36
isolation 158; and rejection 76

jargon 4
joining and not joining 183

kitchen 173
knowledge of grief 21
known stillbirth 33, 38
Kübler-Ross, E. 6

lack of a happy outcome 151
lack of contact 35
lack of engagement 155
lack of experience 154
lack of groups 186
lack of support 155, 158
lack of time 24
lactation 66, 76, 77
language 60
lay support systems 179
learned helplessness 74
legitimacy of mourning 36

legitimate sorrow 95
lesser losses xi
let go 192
limited autonomy 155
limited resources 152
Lindemann, E. 6
living without the dead person 83
lone fatherhood 135
lone twin 102
loss 1; of future 99; of self 35; of
    uniqueness 184
love at first sight 15
Lovell, A. 77
Lovell, H. 77

macho toughness 177
magical thinking 104
making adjustments 176
making contact 112, 181
making time 71
managers' support 159
marital conflict 93
maternal death 129
maternal mortality 129
McHaffie, H.E. 116, 146
meaning of the pregnancy 37
measurement 24
medical sociology 180
medicalisation 180
mementoes 93
memories xi, 34
methodology 25
midwife and maternal death 135
midwife's role 6
midwife's visits 33, 87
midwives' shortcomings 153
miscarriage 23, 41, 93, 209; pain of 42
misgivings 184
morbid atmosphere 184
mortality rate 130
mother with HIV/AIDS 55
mother's anger 152
mourning 2, 67; rituals of 79
multiple pregnancy 101
multiplicity of demands 155
mutual aid 180
mutual benefit 180
mutual support 84, 157
mutuality of experience 192

name of child 202, 205
narcissism 198
narratives 166
natural way 95, 176

negative stress 160
neonatal unit (NNU) 108, 161;
  environment of 121, 126
newborn with a handicap 48
newsletters 193
not moving on 192
nursery 73

obtaining the care that a new mother
  needs 77
occupational denial 139
openness 146
optimal environment 120
organisational factors 154
other social support 73
out of bounds 146
out of place 184
out-of-the-blue approach 182
outside baby 18
overlap 185

packages of care 81
palliative care 159
panacea 27
paradox 140
parental involvement in care 115
Parkes, C.M. 7, 80
passing on information 182
past events 119
pathological grief 10, 79
peer support 156, 162
perfect baby 17
perinatal bereavement counselling 85
perinatal grief scale 94
personal factors 153
personal growth 207
personal implications of research 29
personal loss xi
person-centred counselling 82
photos 67
pitfalls 72
politics 143, 180
post-mortem 72, 110
postnatal bonding 16
postnatal ward 176
prediction 24
pregnancy changes 15
prenatal diagnosis (PND) 45, 46
preparing the parents 114
preparing to face the future 72
primary prevention 161
principles of care 59, 63
professional services 84
professionalism 170

professionals 146
protecting 90, 93
providing time 83
psychoanalytic theory 6
psychodynamic counselling 82
psychosocial support 121
PTSD (post traumatic stress disorder)
  23, 40
public health reform 133

qualitative study 81
questioning 20
quota 71

Rådestad, I. 177
Rajan, L. 71
RCT 65
reactions after the birth 40
realisation 9
realising she is a mother 66
reality of her baby 63
reciprocity 187
recognising baby has been born 66
recognising having had baby 63
recognising 'normal' grief 83
recognising that her baby has died 66
recognition 43
Redshaw, M.E. 112
referrals 86
relationship change 98
relationships 3
religion 60
relinquishment 49, 71
relocating the emotions 83
remembrance service 163
replacement child 201, 204
representations of maternal death 131
representativeness 25
research 20, 64
research ethics committees 27
research needs 31
resolution 9
resource implications 123
end of life decision-making 123
response 25
ritual 3, 35, 61, 67
routinisation 58
'rugger pass' approach 27, 145

safe motherhood 143
sample size 25, 29
SANDS 161, 181
secondary loss 99, 197
secondary prevention 161

security 14
sedation 66
self-help 33, 84, 179
self-referrals 86
self-care 180
self-disclosure 184
self-esteem 184
sense of identification 169
sensitive period 17
separation 14
serial reciprocity 187
setting in which care happens 124
sex 98, 197
sharing emotions 168
sharing grief 51
sibling grief 211
sibling loss 103, 105
siblings 23
SIDS 85
silent miscarriage 41
six week medical check 24
sluice 172
snowball 94
social and staff support 121
social support 12
socio-economic class 184
somatic symptoms 8
spontaneous behaviour 176
spousal loss 179
staff: coping with death 33; reactions 145; room 173; support 145
stages of grieving 6
stillbirth 37
stress 145, 159, 178
structures of meaning 209
subsequent pregnancy 201, 203
substitute carers 135
sudden death 85
supervisor of midwives 140
support 61, 91, 93, 99, 141, 160; long term/short term 73
surface acting 165
survey 167
systematic review 82, 88
systems theory 89

teamwork 141

telling about grieving 72
'tender loving care' (TLC) 155
tentative pregnancy 46
terminal care 162
termination of pregnancy 43; for fetal abnormality 45
terminology 79
tertiary interventions 161
TFC (The Compassionate Friends) 187, 194
timing of pregnancy 199
touch and handling 125
transfer home 32
twenty-four hour presence 87
twins 101

ultra sound 15
unclean status 61
uncomplicated grieving 79
unexpected loss 11
unexpected stillbirth 39
unfinished business 96
unhelpful words 4
unique features 34
unique meaning 208
unnaturalness 146
unpreparedness 151
unprofessional 169
unreality 34
unseen loss 93
untimeliness 35, 146
unwelcome 184

validating feelings 87
vanishing twin 102
vertical transmission 55
voluntary services 84

Walter, T. 6, 192
way of being 82
Westernisation 60
WHO 180
women's movement 180
working environment 155, 160

youth of parents 36